Fines will be charged if items are returned late.
Please return this item on or before the last date shown above.
Online Renewals: www.wlv.ac.uk/lib/myaccount
Telephone Renewals: 01902 321333 or 0845 408 1631

UNIVERSITY OF
WOLVERHAMPTON
KNOWLEDGE • INNOVATION • ENTERPRISE

Harrison Learning Centre
City Campus
University of Wolverhampton
St. Peter's Square
Wolverhampton
WV1 1RH
Telephone: 0845 408 1631
Online Renewals: www.wlv.ac.uk/lib/myaccount

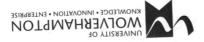

In memory of Che

Expanding Nursing Knowledge

Understanding and researching your own practice

Gary Rolfe
PhD, MA, BSc, RMN, PGCEA

Principal Lecturer, School of Health Studies, University of Portsmouth, UK

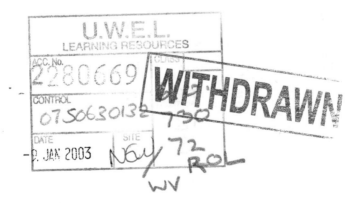
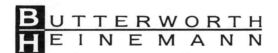

BUTTERWORTH
HEINEMANN

Butterworth-Heinemann
Linacre House, Jordan Hill, Oxford OX2 8DP
225 Wildwood Avenue, Woburn, MA 01801-2041
A division of Reed Educational and Professional Publishing Ltd

℞ A member of the Reed Elsevier plc group

OXFORD   BOSTON   JOHANNESBURG
MELBOURNE   NEW DELHI   SINGAPORE

First published 1998

© Reed Educational and Professional Publishing Ltd 1998

British Library Cataloguing in Publication Data
Rolfe, Gary
    Expanding nursing knowledge: understanding and researching
    your own practice
    1 Nursing – Practice
    I Title
    610.7'3

ISBN 0 7506 3013 2

Library of Congress Cataloguing in Publication Data
Rolfe, Gary
    Expanding nursing knowledge: understanding and researching
    your own practice/Gary Rolfe
        p.   cm.
    Includes bibliographical references and index
    ISBN 0 7506 3013 2
    1 Nursing – Research. I Title
    [DNLM: 1 Nursing Research. 2 Research Design. WY 20.5 R746e 1998]
    RT81.5.R64   97–36320
    610.73'072 – dc21   CIP

Disk manipulation and artwork drawings by David Gregson Associates,
Beccles, Suffolk
Printed and bound in Great Britain by Biddles Ltd., Guildford and King's Lynn

Contents

Preface   vii

PART ONE: UNDERSTANDING YOUR PRACTICE   1

1 Nursing knowledge   7
   Nursing and the scientific paradigm   7
   The limitations of technical rationality   13
   Beyond technical rationality: other ways of knowing   25
   Notes to Chapter 1   37

2 Professional judgement   40
   Developing personal theory   40
   Personal theory and professional judgement   49
   Notes to Chapter 2   63

PART TWO: RESEARCHING YOUR PRACTICE   65

3 A new paradigm for the practitioner–researcher   71
   Towards a new paradigm   71
   Asking practitioner-centred research questions   88
   Methodologies for practitioner-centred research   92
   Summary   99
   Notes to Chapter 3   101

4 Single-case experimental research   102
   Background and rationale   102
   Research questions   103
   Methodology and research design   105
   Data collection methods   116
   Validity and reliability   119
   Data analysis   121
   Summary   124

5 Reflective case-study research   127
   Background and rationale   127
   Research questions   132
   Methodology and research design   135
   Data collection methods   140
   Validity and reliability   158
   Data analysis   162
   Summary   167
   Notes to Chapter 5   168

6 Reflexive action research   171
    Background and rationale   171
    Research questions   176
    Methodology and research design   177
    Data collection methods   189
    Validity and reliability   191
    Data analysis   194
    Summary   195
    Notes to Chapter 6   196

Epilogue: towards a critical community   199

References   206

Index   215

Preface

Two worlds of knowledge

The purpose of this book is to explore ways in which nurses and other health care practitioners can carry out personal research studies into their own practice. This might at first sight appear to be a straightforward issue that hardly warrants a whole book. However, as we shall see, it is far from simple, and the notion of the practitioner–researcher raises a number of complex methodological and practical problems.

Arguably, the root of all of these problems is with the nursing research paradigm itself, which advocates and promotes generalizable scientific knowledge generated by academic researchers who come in to practice areas as outsiders in order to carry out objective research studies. The very notion of nurses subjectively researching their own practice is therefore alien to the dominant research paradigm. Nurses are not expected to tell their own personal stories from their own perspectives, but to bring in outside scientists in order to make objective generalizations which can be applied far beyond the subjects of the study.

The need for this book becomes apparent when we start to examine the kind of knowledge that these academic researchers are interested in. They wish to know about how patients *in general* respond to a particular treatment, not how Mr Jones responded; about what nurses *usually* do in a particular situation, not what nurse Smith did. And they certainly do not want to know about how they as researchers influence the situation they are studying. In fact, they go to great lengths to avoid influencing the situation at all. The idiosyncrasies of individual people get in the way, they introduce unwanted variables into the clinical setting and reduce the external validity or generalizability of the research findings. They must therefore be controlled for, either in the selection of the research sample or in the design of the research itself.

The reason that most researchers avoid studying individuals, including themselves, is because they are interested in a specific kind of knowledge, what the philosopher Karl Popper called 'world 3' knowledge. World 3 knowledge is mostly knowledge about the world in general, and about people in general. It can be found in books, journals and other publicly accessible media, and the most usual way of generating world 3 knowledge is through the scientific method. World 3 knowledge forms the foundation of the science of nursing. In contrast to researchers, practising nurses are becoming more and more concerned with personal knowledge, knowledge about themselves or knowledge which they alone possess. Popper referred to this as 'world 2' knowledge, knowledge which is not in the public domain and probably never will be. Indeed, for many scientists it does not qualify as knowledge at all.

Scientific world 3 knowledge tells us how patients with a certain illness *tend* to respond to a particular treatment, whereas personal world 2 knowledge allows us to look beyond the illness to the person himself. Thus, if nursing is ever to become fully holistic and patient centred rather than disease focused and task oriented, then as well as world 3 knowledge, nurses also need world 2 knowledge, knowledge about themselves, their own clinical practice and their individual patients. Without this personal knowledge, the application of scientific research findings to real-life individual cases will continue to be a hit-and-miss affair based on perceived and often imaginary similarities between patients rather than acknowledging them as unique individuals. Indeed, the gap between theory and practice in nursing is largely the gap between Popper's two worlds: the world of the researcher (world 3) and the world of the practitioner (world 2). The aim of this book is to attempt to unite those worlds.

A guidebook for the practitioner–researcher

In many ways, this book can be seen as a companion to my earlier book (Rolfe, 1996), which was to some extent a manifesto for a new nursing paradigm. As well as presenting a rationale for the new paradigm, that book also described the role of the nurse–practitioner who generated her own knowledge and theory from and for her own practice in a process which I referred to as praxis. However, although providing a number of examples of the paradigm in action, it was essentially a theoretical and rather abstract book.

In contrast, this new work more closely resembles a guidebook whose aim is to enable the nurse–practitioner to fulfil her dual role of knowledge generator and knowledge applier (in fact, the roles cannot be separated, and are two sides of the same coin). Part One examines the sort of knowledge and theory needed for this new paradigm of nursing, and Part Two explores how that knowledge can be acquired. And at the risk of spoiling the ending, I conclude that in order to obtain the sort of knowledge she requires for her practice, the nurse–practitioner has little alternative but to carry out her own research with her own patients in her own clinical area. The nurse–practitioner therefore becomes in this book the practitioner–researcher; if academic researchers are unwilling to tell her story then she must tell it herself.

I stated in the preface to my first book that the finished product was not the book I had intended to write, and that statement applies equally to the book you are now reading. The book I had intended to write was a simple, practical, users' guide for practitioners who wished to research their own practice. However, once I started to write, it quickly became apparent that there were two obstacles to achieving this aim.

First, the methodologies required for researching our own practice seemed to be breaking most of the established rules of the dominant scientific paradigm. Secondly, the kind of knowledge that this sort of research was generating was very different from the knowledge produced by traditional scientific research. Clearly, if I was not to be left open to criticism by more traditional researchers, these two issues would need to be addressed before I could go on to explore the research methods and methodologies themselves.

This book therefore contains not only a fairly extensive theoretical discussion about this new research paradigm and how it differs from the old, but also a whole section on nursing knowledge and what it means to the practitioner who wishes to carry out research into herself and her own practice. It is only after all these issues have been considered that the book can get down to its real business of exploring a variety of research methodologies for the practitioner–researcher.

However, despite having to address these theoretical issues in some depth, I have attempted to remain true to my original intention of producing a practical user's guide for nurses who wish to explore their own practice, and to some extent the discipline of having to delve into the theoretical underpinnings of practitioner–research has produced a more holistic and coherent book than the one I originally intended to write. It is, I hope, rather more substantial than the 'cookbook' approach taken by many traditional research texts, and attempts to guide the reader through a practical examination of the knowledge and theory which informs her clinical decisions as well as providing a detailed rationale for the new research paradigm.

A note on terminology

I continue to struggle with certain problems of terminology, particularly concerning gender. I will therefore follow the conventions of my earlier book and employ the female gender to denote the person of power or authority in any relationship, and the male gender to denote the other. This, of course, means that nurses will usually be referred to by the feminine pronoun (except when I am writing about a nurse in a student–teacher relationship), which introduces the problem of stereotyping all nurses as women. However, until suitable gender-free terminology is developed, I consider this to be the best solution in an imperfect world. I will also employ the conventions of my previous book by using the terms 'patients' and 'nurses' throughout, for which I hope 'clients' and 'consumers' of the health services, and my midwife and health visitor colleagues will forgive me.

You will also have noticed by now that this book is written mostly in the first person singular. This was a deliberate and considered decision which follows from the two main themes of the book: first, the valuing of knowledge which arises from personal experience and reflection; and, secondly, the argument that such knowledge can only be obtained by taking an overtly subjective stance. I have attempted to practise what I preach by employing examples from my own experience, and of course my own personal knowledge can only authentically be recounted in the first person.

Furthermore, this approach to writing is my statement of ownership of the ideas expressed in this book. By writing 'I believe that ...' rather than 'It is considered that ...', I am taking full responsibility for the book's content rather than hiding behind the impersonal passive case. Finally, I believe that the first person is easier on the eye and the brain of the reader than some of the more convoluted alternatives.

Part One

Understanding your practice

This book, like its predecessor (Rolfe, 1996), argues for a shift in the way that the nursing profession defines and organizes itself, that is, for a new nursing paradigm. The term 'paradigm' has been defined and used in many different ways, but for the purpose of this book, I will employ the definition offered by Powers and Knapp (1990) of an organizing framework which contains:

- Concepts, theories, assumptions, beliefs, values and principles that form a way for a discipline to interpret the subject matter with which it is concerned.
- Research methods considered to be best suited to generating knowledge within this frame of reference.
- What is open to investigation – priorities and views on knowledge deficit areas where research and theory building is most needed.
- What is closed to inquiry for a time.

The dominant paradigm of a discipline is therefore extremely powerful in determining the nature of what counts as knowledge, how it is generated and how it is disseminated, as well as the underlying values and beliefs of that discipline. It attempts to provide answers to questions such as: what is nursing knowledge? who owns it? where does it come from? how can we develop it? how does it apply to practice? how can we transmit and disseminate it?

Kuhn (1962) argued that shifts in the dominant paradigm occur suddenly, and arguably the most recent paradigm shift in British nursing is just now coming to fruition with the (sometimes reluctant) acceptance of nursing as an academic discipline. This shift has established a scientific research base for nursing knowledge as well as a 'technocratic' approach to nurse education (Bines, 1992), and stands in stark contrast to the previous practice-based paradigm for generating knowledge and the 'pre-technocratic' model for its dissemination.

Thus, when I trained as a psychiatric nurse in the early 1980s (before the shift to the current paradigm), I served what was in effect an apprenticeship, and my knowledge of nursing grew naturally (if somewhat slowly) out of that process. The vast majority of my time as a student was spent with practising nurses in clinical areas, and the purpose of the occasional two-week taught block in the school of nursing was to consolidate the learning which had taken place 'on the job'. I was taught a certain amount of theory, but it was largely biological and psychiatric theory rather than theory about nursing. Nursing knowledge was something which related first and foremost to practice and not to theory.

In my own field of psychiatric nursing, the swing from practical nursing knowledge to theoretical knowledge (and hence, the first tentative steps towards a paradigm shift) began with the 1982 *Mental Nursing Syllabus*. This was divided into two sections entitled 'Nursing Skills' and 'The Knowledge Base', the latter of which introduced large chunks of sociology and psychology into the curriculum and attempted to construct psychiatric nursing knowledge primarily from the knowledge-bases of disciplines outside of nursing.

This philosophy spread to general nursing with the introduction of *Project 2000* (which was partly based on the 1982 Mental Health Syllabus) in the late 1980s, when we witnessed a sudden influx of sociologists, psychologists and biologists into schools of nursing. This was followed soon after by the integration of those schools into universities and colleges of higher education, accompanied by the promise that nursing was at last becoming a serious academic discipline.

As well as attempting to appropriate relevant knowledge from a variety of other disciplines, nursing was also developing theory and knowledge of its own, both empirically through a growing body of research findings, and also a priori through the construction of theoretical nursing models. This shift in focus from practical to theoretical nursing knowledge was demonstrated in many of the early Project 2000 curricula, where students were subjected to a protracted period of classroom teaching before being allowed into clinical areas to apply what they had learnt.

In the 1990s, however, we are beginning to see a reaction to this scientific, theory-based paradigm of technical rationality. There are growing signs of a shift back in the opposite direction and a formal recognition of nursing knowledge from and for practice, as demonstrated by a growing interest in issues such as reflective practice and clinical supervision. This is to be welcomed, but too often nurses and managers jump on the bandwagon of the latest clinical and educational fads without fully understanding their underlying philosophy or rationale.

By failing to recognize or account for the epistemological foundations of these innovations, reflection becomes just another technique for applying theory to practice, and clinical supervision is seen merely as a tool for helping with caseload management. Although these are important issues, they rather subvert the original aims and intentions of both reflective practice and clinical supervision, which were developed as ways of enabling practitioners to not only take control of their own practice, but also to generate knowledge and theory *from* that practice.

Part One of this book is an attempt to take the idea of practice-based nursing knowledge and theory to its logical conclusions, and that entails challenging much of what nursing currently takes for granted; in effect, it means finding an alternative to the dominant paradigm on which nursing is founded, with its dependence on the traditional scientific method, its hierarchy in which academics and researchers are elevated above practitioners, and its application of generalizable research findings to practice settings.

In challenging the dominant paradigm and formulating a new one, it is therefore necessary to explore critically what nursing knowledge is, how it is generated, and how it is disseminated, and these concerns form the framework for the two parts of this book. The primary concern of Part One is with the nature of nursing knowledge, that is, with epistemology: 'the philosophical theory of knowledge, which seeks to define it, distinguish its principal varieties, identify its sources, and establish its limits' (Bullock *et al.*, 1988).

It begins by outlining the scientific paradigm and the traditional relationship between research, knowledge and theory, and then goes on to examine the application of the scientific paradigm to nursing practice, what Schön (1983) referred to as technical rationality. The limitations of technical rationality are explored, and its influence is associated with the growing gap in nursing between theory and practice.

Part One then looks beyond technical rationality by exploring other forms of knowledge, and attempts to integrate them in a model of professional judgement, which is based on the knowledge that the nurse acquires by reflecting on her own experience. Finally, it looks at how professional judgement is related to the development of nursing practice, and how the nurse who employs her professional judgement to make clinical decisions requires a new paradigm of research which generates knowledge and theory for practice in a way that scientific research is unable to do.

I hope that you will actively participate in this exploration of the epistemology of nursing, and I have included a number of structured breaks along the way for thought and reflection.

REFLECTIVE BREAK

THEORY-BASED AND PRACTICE-BASED KNOWLEDGE

You will find a number of reflective exercises throughout this book. They give you an opportunity to stop and think about what you have read and to apply it to your own work, so please do not skip over them. They also allow you to contribute to the book and to personalize it, and for that reason, space has been provided for you to write directly on to the page. If you own this copy, please do not be afraid to write on it.

Books should be regarded as resources which offer a particular point of view, and just because something is printed in a book, this does not mean that it is the final word on the subject. Feel free to add, subtract and amend. Of course, if this book belongs to someone else or is a library copy, please ignore the above, as I do not want libraries sending me bills for encouraging readers to deface their books!

Many of the reflective exercises in this book can also be used as a basis for group discussions if you are working through them with colleagues.

Now think back to your own nurse training:

- Where did your knowledge come from?

- Was it mainly practice-based or theory-based knowledge?

- How does it differ from the knowledge-base of students you come into contact with now?

- What does this tell you about the way that nurse training has changed?

1

Nursing knowledge

Nursing and the scientific paradigm

The first part of this book is concerned with the nature of nursing knowledge and its implications for practice. Nursing practice, we are informed by the Department of Health (1989), should be based on scientific research, and I shall therefore begin by exploring the philosophy and methods of science. The scientific view of nursing is widespread throughout the discipline, prompting assertions such as: 'nursing is a science and the application of knowledge from that science to the practice of nursing' (Andrews and Roy, 1986). However, while Benner and Wrubel (1989) claimed that nursing research is 'in the tradition of classical seventeenth century science', few nurse theorists would rigorously attempt to apply the traditional 'hard' scientific methods to the generation of nursing knowledge. Rather, there is a general consensus that nursing research should employ the 'soft' methodologies of the social sciences.

Hard and soft science

The difference between the two is neatly summed up by Hughes (1990). The hard sciences, such as physics and chemistry, are characterized by invariable laws of cause and effect, such that effect E *always* follows cause C. Consider, for example, the law of gravity, which states that two bodies will attract one another with a force proportional to their masses and the distance between them, or more simply, that what goes up must (eventually) come down. As a hard scientific law, this does not mean that two bodies *sometimes* attract one another, or that what goes up *usually* comes down, but that it is always and invariably the case.

This is contrasted with the softer social sciences, which are based on the statistical concepts of correlation and probability, where E *usually* follows C. Thus, the sociological relationship between poverty and ill-health does not imply that the poor *always* suffer from illness, but only that it is generally the case, or that the poor usually suffer worse health than the rich.

Even medical research, which prides itself on its scientific under-pinnings, lies at the soft end of the continuum. When medical researchers tell us that smoking causes lung cancer, they do not mean that smoking *always* results in cancer, but that statistically, your chances of developing lung cancer are higher if you smoke than if you do not. Thus, 'while the use of such [soft research] techniques have (sic) resulted in any number of empirical generalizations, none has been so far offered as a causal law' (Hughes, 1990). This statistical or probabilistic nature of knowledge in the soft sciences is important, as we shall see later.

Even at the soft end of the soft science of nursing, however, there is still a healthy respect for the rigours of the scientific method. Denzin (1997) referred to this position as postpositivist, and argued that although it views qualitative research as requiring an alternative para-digm to that of positivism, with its own unique criteria,

> In practice ... this position has often led to the development of a set of criteria that are in agreement with the positivist criteria; they are merely fitted to a naturalistic research context.

Furthermore, Hammersley (1992) noted that those criteria included the generation of formal theory, scientific credibility and generaliz-ability, all strongly positivist values.

Research, knowledge and theory

The scientific paradigm suggests a clear and simple relationship between knowledge and research: scientific research is the application of the methods of science, and the reason for doing research is to generate scientific knowledge. This relationship can be discerned in almost any definition of nursing research, for example: '[research is] an attempt to identify facts, and the relationship between and among facts, by systematic, scientific enquiry in order to increase available knowledge' (Hunt, 1982); 'the primary goal of nursing research is to develop a scientific knowledge base for nursing practice' (Burns and Grove, 1987); 'research is an attempt to increase available knowledge by the discovery of new facts or relationships through systematic enquiry' (Macleod Clark and Hockey, 1989); and '[research is] a systematic approach and a rigorous method with the purpose of generating new knowledge' (International Council of Nurses, 1996).

So the aim of nursing research is to generate knowledge, but what of theory? The relationship between knowledge and theory is rather less well defined, and as Slevin and Basford (1995) have pointed out, the terms are often used synonymously. There is also some confusion, particularly in nursing, between the terms 'theory' and 'model'. Merton (1968) distinguished between grand theory, essentially untestable and composed of abstract concepts in relationship; middle-range theory, composed of less abstract concepts capable of verification by research; and micro-theory, which is usually related to specific research hypotheses or propositions.

The philosopher Karl Popper (1979) argued that the criterion which distinguishes scientific theories from non-scientific ones is the possibility of disproving the former; scientific theories must be open to refutation. We can see, then, that scientific research is not directly concerned with the rather nebulous and unrefutable grand theories and models, but with middle-range and micro-theories, theories which are open to the possibility of being disproved. Slevin and Basford offered a definition of this kind of theory as:

> the description or explanation of phenomena and the relationships between such phenomena ... [which] may go beyond the purely descriptive or explanatory levels, to the level of prediction.
>
> (Slevin and Basford, 1995)

Thus, theory orders knowledge in a descriptive, explanatory or predictive framework. It enables us to employ knowledge in order to describe the world, to explain it, and most importantly, to make predictions about it.

Let us take an example to demonstrate the relationship between scientific research, knowledge and theory (Figure 1.1). In the early seventeenth century, Galileo made extensive systematic observations of the heavens, and from the data collected as a result of this research, he derived the knowledge that the planets often move in erratic and unpredictable ways which could not be accounted for by the then-dominant theory that the stars and the planets revolved around the Earth, which stood at the centre of the universe.

This knowledge was not new; indeed, the Greeks and Romans both attempted to explain the unpredictable movements of the planets with the pre-scientific (and untestable) theory that the planets were gods and could therefore move wherever they wanted. Galileo's theory

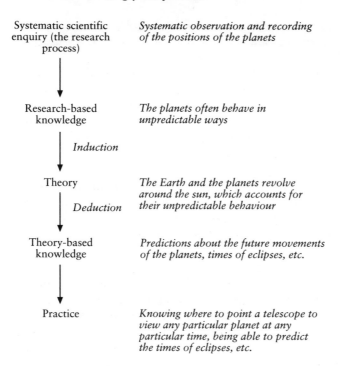

Systematic scientific enquiry (the research process) — *Systematic observation and recording of the positions of the planets*

Research-based knowledge — *The planets often behave in unpredictable ways*

Induction

Theory — *The Earth and the planets revolve around the sun, which accounts for their unpredictable behaviour*

Deduction

Theory-based knowledge — *Predictions about the future movements of the planets, times of eclipses, etc.*

Practice — *Knowing where to point a telescope to view any particular planet at any particular time, being able to predict the times of eclipses, etc.*

Figure 1.1   *Constructing and using a scientific theory.*

(which he borrowed from Copernicus), however, was that the Earth was not in fact the centre of the universe, around which everything else revolved, but was just one of several planets revolving around the sun, and that it was the complex interaction of the rotation of the Earth and the other planets which produced the seemingly haphazard movements of the planets when viewed from the Earth.

From this example, we can see the first function of a scientific theory, which is to describe, explain, or otherwise make sense of existing knowledge. It must be emphasized that a theory is more than just an accumulation of knowledge, and Galileo's theory did not merely collect together all his experiences and observations, which would have constituted a fairly meaningless mass of data. Rather, he built them into a body of theory which was greater then the sum of its parts through a process known as induction.

Induction, or inductive reasoning, is one of the ways that science constructs generalizable, universal theories from finite, limited sets of data; it is a way of arguing from the specific to the general. Galileo did not, and could not, observe every movement of every planet all the time, since such a task is clearly impossible, even in the age of radio telescopes and computers. Rather, he took a *sample* of all the possible data, and reasoned that because the planets moved in a particular fashion whenever he observed them, that they would continue to do so all the time that he was not observing them. He therefore generalized his observations of what happened on specific occasions into a theory of what always happens on all occasions.

A theory gives new meaning to existing knowledge, and therefore results in a shift in our perceptions; it enables, indeed compels, us to see the world in a new light.[1] In Galileo's case, once we think of the Earth and the planets as revolving around the sun, not only does the apparently erratic movement of the planets suddenly make sense, but we find that their movement is not, after all, erratic but that it can be determined with great precision.

This brings us to the second function of a theory, which is to predict what we do not yet know, that is, to generate *new* knowledge. This entails a process known as deduction or deductive reasoning, which is in a sense the opposite of induction. Whereas inductive reasoning takes us from the specific to the general, deductive reasoning takes us from the general back to the specific. Thus, from the general theory that the Earth and the planets moved around the sun, Galileo was able to make specific predictions, for example, of times of eclipses.

Theory, then, not only explains and orders knowledge, but can be employed to construct it, which in turn leads to new theories, and so on. Furthermore, the predictions which arise out of theories serve to test those theories: if the predictions are confirmed, then the theory can continue to be used; if the predicted events do not come about, then the theory is modified or discarded. In Galileo's case, if the planets did not move as he had predicted, then perhaps the Greeks and Romans were right after all, and the planet Mars is indeed a god who rides across the heavens in his chariot throwing lightning bolts! It should be borne in mind, however, that theories can never be confirmed beyond doubt, and that the aim of scientific research is not to prove, but to disprove, a theory.

Scientific theory can also direct and influence practice. In the above example, Galileo's theory not only increased the *knowledge base* of astronomy by accurately predicting the movements of the planets, but it also improved the *practice* of astronomy by telling astronomers exactly where to point their telescopes to view any particular planet at any particular time. Schön (1983) described this relationship between scientific knowledge and practice, where practice is informed and dictated to by science, as 'technical rationality', which he defined as 'the Positivist epistemology of practice'.

Technical rationality nursing

The Department of Health, as we saw at the start of this chapter, suggested that 'all clinical practice should be founded on up-to-date information and research findings' (Department of Health, 1989), that is, it should be based on Schön's model of technical rationality. It would seem appropriate, therefore, to attempt to apply the scientific research process outlined above to the generation of nursing knowledge, theory and practice. Let us take the example, based on research, of what to say to terminally ill patients who ask whether or not they are dying (Figure 1.2).

The first step in generating the scientific knowledge required to answer the question is to systematically collect data by carrying out

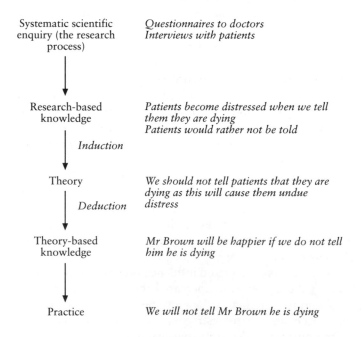

Figure 1.2   *Constructing and using a scientific nursing theory.*

research. For example, we might send out questionnaires to doctors to ask what they find are helpful responses, or conduct interviews with patients to enquire about what they would wish to be told. This enables us to generate the research-based knowledge that, to take a hypothetical example, doctors have found that patients tend to become distressed when we tell them they are dying, or that most patients say that they would rather not be told.

From this knowledge, we can inductively formulate the scientific theory that we should not tell patients that they are dying in order not to cause them undue distress. This theory can then be employed deductively to make predictions about individual situations, for example, that Mr Brown will be happier if we do not tell him that he is dying. The theory can also, of course, be employed to direct practice: thus, because research has shown that patients are better off not knowing that they are dying, we will therefore not tell Mr Brown that he has only two weeks to live.

This, strictly speaking, is the approach that Andrews and Roy (1986) were advocating when they claimed that 'nursing is a science and the application of knowledge from that science to the practice of nursing', and also what the Department of Health meant when it advocated the notion of research-based practice. Now look at the Reflective Break on page 14.

The limitations of technical rationality

There are, in fact, a number of problems when it comes to applying scientific theory to nursing practice. You might recall from earlier that a scientific theory performs two functions: first, it gives order and structure to what we already know; and secondly, it enables us to create new knowledge by making predictions about what we do not yet know. Our scientific nursing theory to some extent achieves the first of these functions by making sense of all our individual pieces of research data about whether we should inform terminally ill patients that they are dying. But what about the second function: are we able to make predictions from our theory? Can we really be sure that our theory will tell us how Mr Brown would want us to respond if he was to ask us whether he was dying?

Similarly, in trying to answer the questions in the Reflective Break on page 14, you might well have made different decisions depending on whether or not you knew the individual patients. In other words, you not only employed scientific research-based knowledge in

REFLECTIVE BREAK

EXPLORING THE LIMITATIONS OF SCIENTIFIC THEORY

Nursing theory based on scientific research predicts that, in general, surgical patients who are given information in advance about their operation will experience less postoperative pain, will require less analgesia and will be discharged home sooner. However, in a few isolated cases, such as for patients with high anxiety levels, giving information can actually make recovery longer and more painful. The problem, however, is that it is very difficult to tell in advance which patients will respond adversely without spending a great deal of time getting to know them as individuals.

You are nursing six patients who you do not know well, and who are due to have surgery in an hour. Do you give them information about their operations?

How did you come to this decision?

You are primary nurse to a group of six patients who you know very well, and who are due to have surgery in an hour. Do you give them information about their operations?

How did you come to this decision?

What do your two decisions tell you about the strengths and limitations of scientific theory in making clinical decisions?

reaching your decision, but also your professional judgement, in the form of your personal knowledge of the patients and your previous clinical experience when it was available to you. Scientific theories are useful for making general statements about how large groups of patients tend to behave or respond, but they cannot reliably predict the behaviour of individuals.

The theory–practice gap

This tension between basing our practice on scientific theory and knowledge on the one hand, and on professional judgement on the other, is nicely illustrated by two seemingly opposing views by the same authors in the same book. On the subject of giving information to patients about to undergo surgery, Bailey and Clarke (1989) wrote:

> From the nursing point of view we can conclude that the provision of procedural and sensory information ... has sufficient research support to justify its routine use ... in surgery.

Elsewhere, however, they claimed that:

> whilst giving factual information is useful, the personal approach means identifying those patients who reveal greater than normal anxiety so that the source can be identified and addressed on an individual basis.

In the first extract, they are advocating the routine application of research-based knowledge; that information should be given to all patients. In the second, however, they are suggesting that professional judgement should be employed on an individual basis; that *not all* patients should be given information. As the philosopher Hans-Georg Gadamer (1996) pointed out:

> What we need to do is to learn to build a bridge over the existing divide between the theoretician who knows the general rule and the person involved in practice who wishes to deal with the unique situation of this patient who is in need of care.

Let us take a second example. Scientific research has provided us with a number of demographic factors which are associated with a risk of committing suicide. For example, we know that there is a statistical correlation between suicide and young men, between suicide and the elderly, and between suicide and the unemployed. We should, then, be able to make predictions based on this scientific knowledge and identify those people at high risk of attempting to kill themselves. However, in practice it is virtually impossible to predict suicide risk on an individual basis, and even the Department of Health, a vigorous advocate of research-based practice, has concluded that:

> All these factors are well-known statistical correlates of suicide and must not be ignored. They do, however, present problems in the day-to-day clinical situation. Many individuals will possess these characteristics yet not commit suicide, and suicide can occur in people of very different characteristics.
>
> (Williams and Morgan, 1994)

Therfore, if we *do* attempt to make our assessments of suicide risk according to the research findings, we run into the problem of 'false positives'. Pallis *et al.* (1984) have pointed out that if we target all those people in high-risk groups, then for each positive identification of a suicidal patient, we will identify another 104 people who fall into the high-risk category but who do not intend to kill themselves. As the artist and poet William Blake put it:

> To generalise is to be an idiot. To particularize is the alone distinction of merit. General knowledge are those that idiots possess.
>
> (Blake, 1808)

It would appear, then, that we have reached the limits of what a scientific nursing theory is able to tell us about practice. In astronomy, the behaviour of the planets is regular and predictable once we have discovered the theory which governs or explains their movements, but even in the hard sciences we can never be *absolutely* certain. The eighteenth century philosopher David Hume pointed out the 'problem of induction', that theories are based on a finite number of individual observations and therefore our observations of the behaviour of the planets in the past gives us no guarantee that they will continue to behave in the same way in the future.

Nevertheless, in the hard sciences we have reasonable grounds to suppose that the future will resemble the past, unlike in nursing, where the behaviour of our individual patients is far from predictable. Our nursing theory might be able to tell us the likelihood or probability that Mr Brown would not wish to be told that he is dying, but it can never tell us with any degree of certainty how he would *actually* respond to the news. Equally, the theory that most patients benefit from being given information about their operations can never reliably tell us how well any individual patient will recover postoperatively, nor can the theory that suicide is related to unemployment or age tell us which of our patients are likely to attempt to kill themselves. It would appear, then, that Blake was right: when it comes to individual cases, general knowledge alone does result in a form of idiocy.

This uncertainty about how any particular individual would respond to nursing interventions based on scientific theory is referred to as the theory–practice gap; the gap between what scientific theory says ought to happen in general, and what actually happens in any individual case. It is also, as Schön pointed out, the gap between 'pure' science and 'applied' technology, between the researcher-scientist and the nurse-technician. As Greenwood pointed out:

> In the evolution of every profession there emerges the researcher-theoretician whose role is that of scientific investigation and theoretical systematization. In technological professions, a division of labor thereby evolves between the theory-oriented and the practice oriented person.
>
> (Greenwood, 1966)

Furthermore, it is a hierarchical split, with the academic researcher usually having more status, power and salary than her practice-based nursing colleague. As the educationalist John Elliott pointed out, the power relationship is blind to the research methods employed:

> Whether the techniques generate psychometric measures, ethnographies or grounded theories does not matter. They are all symbolic of the power of the researcher to define valid knowledge.
>
> (Elliott, 1991)

Practising nurses might well be involved in research, but the extent of their involvement will probably be to 'facilitate or assist with data collection for nursing and other health-related research projects being undertaken in their work setting' (International Council of Nurses, 1996), that is, as research assistants. Their main role, however, is to implement the findings of academics. Scientific theory is disseminated down the hierarchy from researcher to practitioner by means of lectures, conferences and academic papers, which are expected to be accepted and implemented as 'research-based practice'. As Pryjmachuk (1996) pointed out:

> It is the theories of the pure scientists that dictate the actions of those in practice, the applied scientists. Though the relationship between theory and practice appears to exist, it seems somewhat unidirectional in nature.

And as Elliott (1991) added, 'theory for [practitioners] is simply the product of power exercised through the mastery of a specialized body of technique'. This unidirectional power relationship (which was explored in Figures 1.1 and 1.2) is illustrated in simplified form in Figure 1.3.

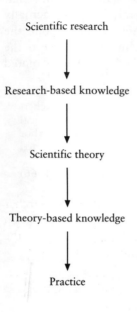

Scientific research

Research-based knowledge

Scientific theory

Theory-based knowledge

Practice

Figure 1.3   *The relationship between scientific research and nursing practice.*

Theoreticians and academics tell us that the theory–practice gap is a result of theory either not being read by practitioners, not being understood when it is read, or else not being properly applied to practice. Thus:

> the blame for the continuation of traditional practices, which research has shown should be changed, cannot be laid at the door of that research. Rather the fault is either one of communication of findings, or of inertia to change.
>
> (Gibbings, 1993)

However, we can see that even if the findings from research are constantly and consistently applied, it will not result in better, more spontaneous, individualized care, but in mechanical, task-centred, uniform practice which does not address the unique individual needs of our unique individual patients. As Stenhouse (1984b) pointed out:

> You don't need a doctor at all if all he is going to give you is a treatment laid down by the State or suggested by his professor without bothering to examine you and make a diagnosis.

Practice based solely on the research findings of others is not enough. Rather, as Gadamer (1996) noted:

> Once science has provided doctors with the general laws, causal mechanisms and principles, they must still discover what is the right thing to do in each particular case, and this is something which hardly seems to be predictable or knowable in advance.

And the same, of course, is true of nurses.

Macro theory and micro practice

In order to understand why the application of knowledge and theory generated from scientific research does not readily translate into safe and effective individualized nursing practice, we must examine in more detail exactly what scientific research *does* tell us. It must be remembered that the research on which nursing theory is built derives largely from the positivist social science paradigm, and occasionally from medical research, and as such, it relies heavily on statistical significance for its external validity or generalizability.

Even qualitative research usually seeks to generalize from a sample to a population, albeit from an often very small sample. The standard data analysis method of categorizing qualitative data into themes and constructs is an attempt to find commonalities across the members of the sample, and by induction, across the whole population which they represent. Thus, when the *Report of the Taskforce on the Strategy for Research in Nursing, Midwifery and Health Visiting* called for 'rigorous and systematic enquiry ... designed to lead to generalizable contributions to knowledge' (Department of Health, 1993), it was calling for research which attempted to make general statements about large populations based on studies conducted with samples representative of those populations.

This approach to research has served nursing well in the past, when the nurse's role was largely task centred. Faced with the prospect of having to give 20 bed-baths in a morning, it is very helpful to know what research has found to be the quickest and most effective method for carrying out that particular task in the majority of cases. However, in these days of primary nursing we are more interested in the personal and unique needs of our individual patients, and there are a number of reasons why scientific, research-based knowledge and theory is woefully inadequate for informing us of those unique and individual needs.

Most of the reasons are concerned with the micro and macro levels at which scientific research operates. This distinction is fairly clear in the social sciences, where research is usually trying to make predictions and offer explanations on a macro level. Thus, an opinion poll of voting intention will attempt to predict how the population as a whole intends to vote, but will tell us nothing about how those findings apply on a micro level. The finding that 75 per cent of the population intends to vote Labour and 25 per cent intends to vote Conservative, might, at first glance, seem to indicate that there is a three in four chance that Mr Smith will vote Labour, but in fact, *nothing whatsoever* can be inferred from the poll about Mr Smith's particular voting intentions.

In order to understand why, it is necessary to examine exactly what the findings from statistically based research *do* tell us. They tell us that if we choose a member of the population at random, there is only one chance in four that we will choose a Conservative voter. But that is very different from supposing that the individual we have chosen has a one in four chance of voting Conservative.

Let us say, for example, that we have chosen Mr Smith, a lifelong Conservative voter who happens to be standing as a Conservative candidate at the forthcoming election. The chances of Mr Smith voting Conservative are certainly not one in four, but probably closer to 999 in 1000. Now let us imagine instead that we chose Mrs Brown, another lifelong Conservative voter who is thinking of changing her voting habits but cannot decide between the two main parties. The chances of Mrs Brown voting Conservative are probably about one in two, or evens. For each person that we randomly choose, there will be a different probability of them voting Conservative, even though the probability of choosing a Conservative voter remains at one chance in four.

People are unique individuals, and macro statistics simply do not apply. As the poet W.H. Auden said: 'as persons, we are incomparable, unclassifiable, uncountable, irreplaceable' (Auden, 1967). Thus, from the findings of our opinion poll, we can estimate the probability of randomly selecting a Conservative voter, but we cannot estimate the probability of any individual person voting Conservative.

Our opinion poll merely tells us that, in any population represented by the sample, roughly three-quarters of people will vote Labour, and one quarter will vote Conservative, and gives us no indication at all about which category Mr Smith, Mrs Brown, or any other individual for that matter, will fall into. For the social scientist, this is not a problem because she is only interested in voting intentions at the macro level; she wishes to know who will win the election rather than how any particular member of the electorate will vote.

Although not so obvious, the same applies to much research in the hard sciences. When an engineer uses research findings to predict the amount by which a piece of steel will expand when heated to a certain temperature, it might seem that she is dealing in certainties, but in fact, she is making a statistical prediction based on the uncertain behaviour of a large number of component individuals in much the same way as the social scientist does when she attempts to predict voting behaviour.

Rather than working with a society made up of large numbers of individual people, however, the engineer is working with a piece of steel made up of a large number of atoms. As the steel gets hot, the particles which make up the atoms start to move around in erratic ways which, as the physicist Werner Heisenberg pointed out, are not only unpredictable but unmeasurable. Thus, the engineer can say nothing about the behaviour on a micro level of any individual atom, but can predict with great accuracy on a macro level how the atoms which make up the piece of steel will behave *en masse*, and it is the concerted movements of these millions of individual atoms that cause the metal to expand.

Carey (1995) gave another example of how, at a micro level, familiar and predictable phenomena turn out to be composed of unpredictable individual components:

> Everyone knows that light is partially reflected from some surfaces – glass, for example. If you have a lamp in your room in daytime, and look out of the window, you can see things outside plus a dim reflection of your lamp. The fact that the lamp is partially reflected means that some photons (light particles) are bounced back by the electrons in the glass, while others pass through. Experiment shows that for every 100 photons an average of 4 bounce back, 96 go through. No one knows why. No one knows how a photon "makes up its mind" which course to follow. No one can predict which course a given photon will opt for. Science can only work out the percentage probability.

Social scientists, physicists and nurses all rely on research which provides them with 'percentage probability'. The nurse, however, unlike the social scientist or the engineer, is working on a micro level with individuals rather than with homogeneous groups, and suffers the same problems as the social scientist who tries to apply her research findings to an individual voter, or the engineer who tries to predict the movements of an individual atom or photon. She finds herself in the realms of probability where she can state the statistical likelihood that nine out of her ten patients will respond to a given nursing intervention, but can say nothing about a particular individual with any degree of certainty.

This can be clearly seen in the earlier example of suicide risk assessment. If a psychiatric nurse attempts to apply the research-based theory of an association between suicide and unemployment by targeting her unemployed patients for specialized care, she will quickly find that she has not necessarily identified those of her patients who are at increased risk. There will probably be suicidal patients who are not unemployed, and there will certainly be unemployed patients who are not suicidal. A simple link between a general theory and a particular patient is just not feasible.

Much of the difficulty in trying to apply macro research to micro practice lies in the related problems of sampling and generalizability. Clinical psychologists Barlow and Hersen (1984) have pointed out that generalizability in clinical research is a complex issue. In order to make broad statements about particular treatment options to a wide population, we must consider not only the extent to which we can generalize to other patients, but also to other nurses and other clinical settings. This entails selecting a very heterogeneous sample which includes members representing or displaying a wide range of variables, and which necessarily implies high intersubject variability; in other words, in order to ensure that all the relevant variables are included, the subjects will need to be very different from one another.

However, a highly heterogeneous sample presents three problems. First, it is very difficult to achieve, and requires access to an enormous and varied population from which to sample. Secondly, significant findings tend to become lost in the data, a phenomenon known as a type II error. A good example of this is in the field of psychotherapy, where research findings from a number of studies collated by Eysenck (1965) appeared to indicate that treatment had no significant effect on outcome. However, because the sample was so heterogeneous, it was found on re-analysing the data that within the sample there was a group of patients who improved with treatment and another group who got worse, and that these two groups cancelled one another out (Bergin, 1966).[2] Psychotherapy therefore *does* have an effect, but it is in danger of being overlooked if the research sample is too heterogeneous.

Thirdly, the more heterogeneous the sample becomes, that is, the greater the population that it tries to emulate, the less relevance the findings have to any individual patient. Thus:

> Ten patients, homogenous for obsessive-compulsive neurosis, may bring entirely different histories, personality variables, and environmental situations to the treatment setting and will respond in varying ways to treatment. That is, some patients will improve and others will not. The average response, however, will not represent the performance of any individual in the group.
>
> (Barlow and Hersen, 1984)

In order to produce findings that can be applied to a particular patient, the sample from which the findings were taken must resemble that patient in all the relevant variables. But if we select a homogeneous sample based on the characteristics of one patient, then the findings are not generalizable to a wider population.

There is also an ethical reason why scientific research-based knowledge and theory is inadequate for nursing practice, and this has been explored in depth by the educationalist Lawrence Stenhouse. Stenhouse was writing about scientific research in the teaching profession, but his insights are just as relevant to nursing. He used the comparison between farming and gardening to demonstrate his argument, pointing out that the so-called 'psycho-statistical paradigm' favoured by the technical rationality model originated in agriculture, where it was developed by the statistician R.A. Fisher to evaluate the effects of different growing conditions on identical fields of crops. By comparing the crop yield between the 'control' and the 'experimental' fields, it is possible to make research-based decisions on the relative merits of, say, two different fertilizers. Therefore:

> A measure of gross yield is an appropriate basis on which to select a crop treatment in large-scale farming, where a standardized procedure in which some plants do not thrive is more acceptable than a diagnostic cultivation of each plant individually.
>
> (Stenhouse, 1979a).

In other words, farmers accept that in any standardized procedure there will be some casualties; some plants will not respond to any particular treatment and will die. The aim, however, is to maximize the yield, to find the treatment which produces the best crop regardless of casualties. Van Manen (1990) identified the same ethos in the social sciences, where 'actions and interventions, like exercises, are seen as repeatable; while subjects and samples, like soldiers, are replaceable'.

In nursing, however, this is a totally unacceptable approach: we cannot nurse according to the ethical principle of the greatest good for the greatest number; we cannot base our working practice on research findings which provide the best *overall* care at the expense of a minority of patients who do worse than they would with an alternative form of treatment. Unlike the farmer, for whom it is impractical to treat each ear of wheat as an individual, we *must* vary the treatment given to each of our patients. The nurse, then, is more like a gardener who treats different plants differently, maximizing the treatment for each individual, and who 'must diagnose before he prescribes and then vary the prescription. The agricultural model assumes the same prescription for all' (Stenhouse, 1979a).

Clearly, then, from the perspective of primary, holistic, individualized nursing, there are a number of problems with the scientific technical rationality paradigm of research-based practice. First, as we saw from Figure 1.3, scientific research is theory oriented; the purpose of research is to generate or test theory, which is then applied to practice. This establishes a gap between the theoreticians and researchers whose job it is to develop and disseminate nursing theory, and the practitioners whose job it is to implement it.

Secondly, scientific research, and hence scientific theory, is built on a macro, statistical foundation which generalizes to whole populations rather than saying anything specific about individual patients. This sets up a gap between what research says should happen in the majority of cases and what actually does happen on an individual, interpersonal level.

Thirdly, this technical rationality paradigm does not reflect the humanistic, person-centred approach that many nurses are now espousing, but treats individuals as components of some greater whole, as a field of wheat rather than as individual plants. Or, to use a different metaphor, technical rationality is 'dehumanizing the process of nursing by drawing an analogy between a human being and a machine' (Aggleton and Chalmers, 1986).

Fourthly, it establishes an elitist system in which the roles of researcher and theory generator are reserved for a chosen few. Thus, in the view of the Department of Health (1995), 'research, done properly, is a highly professional and specialist activity and not suited to every practitioner; but every practitioner needs to be involved in using the results of research'.

The unquestioning implementation by practitioners of knowledge based on scientific research findings has therefore not always led to improved practice, but to a gap between macro, scientific, research-based knowledge and theory on the one hand, and micro, personal, experience-based practice on the other. Many nurses have had first-hand experience of this theory-practice gap such that:

> not all nurses who engage in patient care fully accept the arguments for research-based practice. Many do not feel that research necessarily has relevance to their own work and fail to see a role for themselves in the development of practice through research. Research, for a variety of reasons, has not always addressed the concerns of clinical nurses and frequently does not produce the kind of reliable guide to practice that practitioners require.
>
> (MacGuire, 1991)

This dissatisfaction with research-based practice is also felt in other health-care professions. The clinical psychologist Matarazzo claimed that:

> Even after 15 years, few of my research findings affect my practice. Psychological science *per se* doesn't guide me one bit. I still read avidly but this is of little direct practical help. My clinical experience is the only thing that has helped me in my practice to date.
>
> (cited in Bergin and Strupp, 1972)

Furthermore, a series of surveys summarized by Cohen (1976) indicated that 40 per cent of mental health professionals thought that no research exists that is relevant to practice, and the remainder believed that less than 20 per cent of research articles have any applicability to professional settings.

The kind of knowledge generated by traditional scientific research does not appear to have very much direct relevance for practitioners. But if practice-based knowledge does not come from scientific research, then where does it come from? Or, to paraphrase the sociologist Garfinkel: if nursing practice is the answer, what is the question? Now look at the Reflective Break on page 26.

Beyond technical rationality: other ways of knowing

In order to practice effectively and ethically, nurses must look beyond scientific knowledge and theory, and it is therefore necessary to explore the wider epistemology of nursing. What is required is a form of knowledge that will 'articulate … the basic problems we wish to solve, and … propose and critically assess possible solutions'

REFLECTIVE BREAK

IDENTIFYING MY OWN KNOWLEGE

Table 1.1 below has four columns. In the first column, write down ten things (or as many as you can fit on the page) that you know about nursing, ten 'pieces of knowledge' that you feel you possess. Then, in the second column, write down how you know them, for example, from personal experience or from reading a research report. Finally, in the third column, give each piece of knowledge a score between 1 and 4 for how confident you feel that you really do know it, where:

    1 = not at all confident
    2 = a bit confident
    3 = fairly confident
    4 = absolutely confident

Leave the last column empty for now. We will return to this table later in the book.

Table 1.1

What I know about nursing	How I know it	How confident I am that I know it	What kind of knowledge is it?
1			
2			
3			
4			
5			
6			
7			
8			
9			
10			

(Maxwell, 1984). Traditionally, however, nursing has largely followed the example of the natural and social sciences in its consideration of what knowledge is: like most other sciences, it has either not seen epistemology as an issue of importance, with neither *Baillière's Encyclopaedic Dictionary of Nursing and Health Care* (Weller, 1989) nor *A Dictionary of Nursing Theory and Research* (Powers and Knapp, 1995) having entries under 'knowledge'; or else, as we have seen, it has restricted itself to scientific knowledge.

Indeed, many academics are unable or unwilling to conceptualize any alternatives to scientific research-based knowledge. Hicks (1996), for example, talks of moving from practice based on ritual, that is, on intuition, assumption and tradition, to research-based practice, as if these were the only two options. Nurse researchers have thus generally taken for granted that we all understand and mean much the same thing when we talk about knowledge, and that we all go about developing or increasing it in much the same way.

Knowing how and knowing that

One of the first nurse academics to look beyond scientific research and to consider seriously the nature and importance of practical nursing knowledge, and probably the person whose work has done most to stimulate debate in this area, was Patricia Benner with the publication in 1984 of her book *From Novice to Expert*. Benner employed the terminology of the philosopher Gilbert Ryle in suggesting two kinds of knowledge: 'knowing that' and 'knowing how'. For Ryle (1963) 'knowing that' corresponded to traditional theoretical knowledge, for example, knowing *that* bereaved people generally progress through a number of stages of grieving. In contrast, 'knowing how' corresponded to practical knowledge, for example, knowing how to counsel a grieving person. A number of other nurse theorists have also written about nursing knowledge, most notably Barbara Carper, who suggested four 'fundamental patterns of knowing', namely empirics, ethics, personal knowledge and aesthetics (Carper, 1992).

Schön developed the concept of 'knowing how' further with his notion of knowing-in-action, of knowledge embedded in practice, such that:

> I shall use *knowing-in-action* to refer to the sorts of knowledge we reveal in our intelligent action – publicly observable, physical performances like riding a bicycle and private observations like instant

analysis of a balance sheet. In both cases, the knowing is *in* the action. We reveal it by our spontaneous, skilful execution of the performance; and we are characteristically unable to make it verbally explicit.

(Schön, 1987)

This knowing-in-action has all the qualities of what Polanyi (1962) had some years earlier described as tacit knowledge, personal knowledge which we all posses but find difficult to put into words.

The concept of practical knowledge that cannot be put into words has been recognized for a very long time, and was perfectly illustrated by the ancient Chinese story of a wheelwright who ridiculed the scholarly books which his master was reading, claiming that they were 'the dregs and scum of dead men'. When asked to defend this statement, he argued that all that was worth knowing was unable to be expressed in words and therefore died with the knower. That which could be expressed in words, and which subsequently found its way into books, was not worth knowing and could be dismissed as the dregs of true knowledge.

Applying this argument to himself, the wheelwright described his professional knowledge:

> In making a wheel, if you work too slowly, you can't make it firm; if you work too fast, the spokes won't fit in. You must go neither too slowly nor too fast. There must be co-ordination of mind and hand. Words cannot explain what it is, but there is some mysterious art herein. I cannot teach it to my son; nor can he learn it from me. Consequently, though seventy years of age, I am still making wheels in my old age.
>
> (Chuang Tzu, trans. Giles, 1926)

This practical, tacit knowledge therefore cannot be transmitted to others: 'words cannot explain what it is'. You can only learn to be a wheelwright (or, indeed, a nurse) by *being* one, by serving some sort of apprenticeship. Now look at the Reflective Break on page 29.

Benner was particularly interested in this notion of tacit knowledge, which she saw as the hallmark of expert practice. For Benner, the first step towards becoming an expert was to recognize and employ paradigm cases, particular experiences which are powerful enough to stand out as exemplars of practice. These paradigm cases are neither practical knowing how nor theoretical knowing that, but 'a hybrid between naive practical knowledge and unrefined theoretical knowledge'. Furthermore, many of them are too complex to be transmitted to other people, and therefore represent a store of personal experiential knowledge of individual cases and clinical situations.

REFLECTIVE BREAK

EXPLORING TACIT KNOWLEDGE

Here is an excerpt from an instruction manual for operating a video recorder:

Press **menu**. The **main menu** will appear on the TV screen.
Prest **set** – once to select the **timer rec set** menu.
Press **enter** to select the **timer** screen.
Select the next availble timer position by pressing **set +** or **–**, then press **enter**.

Now try to write some similar instructions for riding a bicycle. You might want to explain how to stop yourself falling off when you are pedalling slowly, how you correct your balance when you start to wobble, or how far over you need to lean when you are turning a corner. Try to be as technically precise as possible.

Most people find it quite difficult to express in words exactly what they do when riding a bicycle. Write down why you think it is that some forms of knowing how are easy to describe, whereas others, such as knowing how to ride a bicycle, are very difficult.

Although these individual paradigm cases might be useful if the nurse encounters a similar situation, they are more effective when collected together. Thus:

> expert nurses develop clusters of paradigm cases around different patient care issues so that they approach a patient care situation using past concrete situations much as a researcher uses a paradigm.
>
> (Benner, 1984)

For Benner, then, expertise develops as the practitioner begins to accumulate many similar instances of personal clinical experiences about particular care issues and formulates them into a body of experiential knowledge which is generalizable to other situations.[3] Benner (1984) referred to the application of experiential knowledge as 'intuitive grasp', which 'is available only in situations where a deep background understanding of the situation exists'.

Knowledge from experience

This intuitive grasp of a situation which an expert appears to possess can appear deceptively simple. The apparent simplicity of expertise is illustrated by the story of a plumber who was called out to a house to repair a central heating boiler which had broken down. After asking one or two simple questions and carefully examining the boiler and the radiators, she took out a size 18 ring spanner and gave one of the pipes a sharp blow half an inch before it joined another pipe, waited for 30 seconds, and then hit it again, a little harder this time. The central heating system immediately burst into life, and the plumber asked for £100 for her services. The householders were puzzled and rather angry that a plumber should charge £100 simply for hitting a pipe with a spanner, and demanded an itemized bill. Two days later, the following bill arrived in the post:

Hitting the central heating pipe with a spanner	£1
Knowing how, when and where to hit it	£99
Total	£100

Clearly, a great deal of expertise went into knowing exactly how, when and where to hit the pipe. As well as a thorough scientific knowledge of fluid mechanics, the plumber also drew on her accumulated store of similar situations and, by asking one or two pertinent questions along with a careful inspection, obtained an understanding of this particular problem. She was then able to hit the pipe in precisely the right way, at precisely the right moment, and in precisely the right place. However, if asked to explain exactly how she knew what to do, she would probably not be able to, and would claim instead that she 'just knew', or that it was something to do with experience.

This same model of expertise can be applied to any practical discipline, including nursing. Therefore, as well as categorizing nursing knowledge according to whether it is practical knowing how or theoretical knowing that, we can also divide it into the three categories of:

- Scientific knowledge, for example, of fluid mechanics or of demographic factors associated with suicide, which exists in books and journals, and which is largely the work of researchers and theoreticians.
- Experiential knowledge, which is Benner's 'clusters of paradigm cases' around particular practice issues, built up over time, and which exists largely in the head of the nurse (or plumber!) from whose experience it derives.
- Personal knowledge, which is knowledge or experience of unique individual clinical situations with individual patients, or indeed, of unique individual central heating systems.

Yet another way of distinguishing between different forms of knowledge was suggested by the philosopher Karl Popper, who made the distinction between 'world 2' knowledge and 'world 3' knowledge. World 2 is the world of our conscious experiences, and contains personal, subjective, organismic knowledge, whereas world 3 is 'the world of the logical *contents* of books, libraries, computer memories, and suchlike' (Popper, 1979, his emphasis), that is, of public, objective knowledge. According to Popper's distinction, world 3 includes scientific knowledge and any experiential knowledge that is written down and made publicly accessible, and world 2 includes the personal and experiential knowledge which we carry around in our heads, including all of our tacit knowledge which we are unable to verbalize.[4]

A typology of nursing knowledge

By combining these different ways of categorizing knowledge, we can construct a typology with six forms of knowing (Table 1.2).

Table 1.2   A typology of nursing knowledge

	Theoretical knowledge (knowing that)	Practical knowledge (knowing how)
Scientific (world 3) knowledge	Things I know which I discovered from books and journals through the media or from a lecture	Things I can do which I learnt from books, from instructions or for which I follow a set of procedures
Experiential (world 2 or 3) knowledge	Things I know which I discovered from my own experience or which I worked out for myself	Things I can do which I worked out for myself, based on my own experiences, and which are sometimes difficult to put into words
Personal (world 2) knowledge	Things I know which relate to specific situations or particular patients which I discovered from my experience or worked out for myself	Things I can do which relate to specific situations or particular patients, and which are sometimes difficult to put into words

Scientific theoretical knowledge is all the things I know which I have discovered from books and journals, through other media, or from lectures, and consists of the body of public, accessible, theoretical knowledge of the discipline. To take an example from my own practice of teaching, scientific theoretical knowledge includes psychological theories of learning and philosophies of curriculum design, as well as individual research studies on, say, the effect of class size on student performance. In nursing, most of what we read in academic journals and textbooks is scientific theoretical knowledge.

Scientific practical knowledge is all the things I can do which I have learnt from books, from instructions, or for which I follow a set of procedures, and which in these days of research-based practice, is derived mainly from scientific theoretical knowledge. For example, in my discipline it includes how to set up an overhead projector according to the instructions, the most effective way (based on research findings) of evaluating a course, or the procedure to follow when counselling a student. Most nursing guidelines and procedures are nowadays based on research and are therefore a form of scientific practical knowledge. Indeed, the International Council of Nurses (1996) recommended the writing and publication of 'clinical practice guidelines' as one of the primary means of turning research into practice.

Experiential theoretical knowledge is all the things I know which I have discovered from my own experiences or which I have worked out for myself. This knowledge cannot be described as scientific, since it has not arisen from scientific research, but it is nevertheless generalizable to other similar cases, and has the potential to become public, world 3 knowledge if it is published or otherwise disseminated. It includes my own theories of learning derived from my experience as a lecturer, my own philosophy of curriculum design, and my own views on the effect of class size on student performance based on my experience of teaching classes of various sizes. In nursing, your own theories about, for example, the importance of touch, based on your own experiences, constitutes experiential theoretical knowledge.

Experiential practical knowledge is all the things I can do which I have worked out for myself, based on my own experiences, and which are often difficult to put into words. Again, this knowledge is generalizable to other similar situations, and often comprises what Benner termed clusters of paradigm cases. It includes being able to fix an overhead projector with a piece of chewing gum, the *actual* most effective way I have found to evaluate a course (despite what the research says), and my own particular method of counselling students. In nursing, the way that you touch patients therapeutically, based on your own theories of touch, is experiential practical knowledge.

Personal theoretical knowledge is all the things I know which relate to specific situations or particular individuals which I have discovered from my own personal experience or worked out for myself. This knowledge can be said to be personal in two ways: it is personal to me as the knower, that is, known only to me; and it is knowledge of individual persons or situations rather than of generalizable clusters of paradigm cases, and includes knowledge of myself. These individual items of personal knowledge are often the building blocks for experiential knowledge, and include what I know about my personal tutees as individual people, and what I know about myself in relation to my work, for example, that I write to deadlines and will only start on a writing project the day before it is due to be submitted. In nursing, much personal theoretical knowledge consists of the things you know about individual patients, including their diagnoses, their particular likes and dislikes, and other social, psychological and medical knowledge.

Personal practical knowledge, finally, is the things I can do which relate to specific situations or particular individuals and which are sometimes difficult to put into words, including what Benner referred to as individual paradigm cases. This includes the ability to hit a particular overhead projector in a certain place in order to make it work, and knowing how to deal with the reaction of a particular individual student who is told that he has failed an assignment. In nursing, much personal practical knowledge is derived from the therapeutic relationships which you have with your patients, and is knowledge of how to respond to them as unique individuals.

We can now see why it was far easier to describe the practical knowledge involved in operating a video recorder than it was to describe the practical knowledge involved in riding a bicycle. Although they are both types of know-how, they are nevertheless different. The knowledge of how to operate a video recorder is scientific practical knowledge, derived from the scientific theoretical knowledge of how a video recorder works, and as such, is fairly easy (although sometimes technical and longwinded) to put into words.

The knowledge of how to ride a bicycle, on the other hand, is experiential practical knowledge, knowledge which I have worked out for myself from my own experiences, and which I have probably never been called upon to try to express in words. Indeed, it is *impossible* to express in words since it 'is not stored in the mind as sets of theoretical propositions, but as a reflectively processed repertoire of cases' (Elliott, 1991). It is what Popper referred to as organismic knowledge, knowledge that is embedded in me as a person rather than knowledge which I have taken from books. Now look at the Reflective Break on page 35.

Knowledge for expertise

The importance of experiential knowledge for nursing has been high-lighted by Benner, who studied the different ways that nurses make clinical decisions. She described the attempt to base our practice purely on scientific knowledge, whether it be knowing how or

REFLECTIVE BREAK

RECOGNIZING DIFFERENT KINDS OF KNOWLEDGE

On the next page is an empty table similar to Table 1.2. Fill in each box with an example from your own practice, e.g. in the top left hand box, write in a piece of your own scientific theoretical knowledge. Use Table 1.2 and the examples I gave earlier from my own practice to help.

Do that now.

Having filled in the table, think about and write down your answers to the following questions:

● Which box(es) did you find the most difficult to complete?

● Why was that?

● Which kind(s) of knowledge do you think the nursing profession values the most?

● Why?

● Which kind(s) of knoweldge do you find the most useful for your own practice?

● Why?

● Which kind(s) of knowledge do you find the least useful?

● Why?

● What do your answers to these questions tell you about the different kinds of nursing knowledge?

Table 1.3

	Theoretical knowledge (knowing that)	Practical knowledge (knowing how)
Scientific (world 3) knowledge		
Experiential (world 2 or 3) knowledge		
Personal (world 2) knowledge		

knowing that, as novice practice. Novices nurse 'by the book', applying what research tells them is the most effective intervention in any situation. As she pointed out:

> The rule-governed behaviour typical of the novice is extremely limited and inflexible. The heart of the difficulty lies in the fact that since novices have no experience of the situation they face, they must be given rules to guide their performance. But following rules legislates *against* successful performance because the rules cannot tell them the most relevant tasks to perform in an actual situation.
>
> (Benner, 1984)

Or taking the cycling analogy a step further: 'Let formal models ... be regarded as training wheels, essential for the first safe rides, unnecessary and limiting once replaced by greater skill' (Gordon, 1984). Novice nurses lack experience, and are therefore forced to base their practice on rules and procedures which are derived mainly from scientific theory and research. However, theory based on scientific knowledge cannot predict how individual patients will respond, and is a major contributory factor to the theory–practice gap. Benner's expert nurses, as we have already seen, are far more likely to make decisions based on their accumulated store of paradigm cases, that is, on their experiential knowledge, falling back on scientific knowledge only when they are confronted with a totally new situation, or to support their experiential knowledge.

In contrast to Benner's focus on *experiential* knowledge as the basis of intuitive grasp, a grounded theory study conducted by Radwin (1995) concluded that *personal* knowledge, what she referred to as 'knowing the patient', was the most important component of expertise, with experiential knowledge, or 'matching a pattern' being less therapeutic and only used when personal knowledge was lacking.

Both of these views would seem to offer only a partial explanation of how experts function, and Clarke *et al.* (1996) maintained that expert practitioners must 'draw on both their knowledge of the context in which they are working and their non-contextualized professional knowledge'. Expert clinical decisions require a combination of all three types of knowledge. Scientific knowledge without experiential or personal knowledge results in Benner's novice practice, and is characterized by newly qualified nurses who work 'by the book'. Experiential and personal knowledge without scientific knowledge, on the other hand, is exemplified by the experienced care assistant, who usually knows the right thing to do, but cannot explain or justify her decisions, and is lost when placed in a novel clinical situation. But as Gadamer (1996) pointed out:

> Among all the sciences concerned with nature the science of medicine is the one which can never be understood entirely as a technology, precisely because it invariably experiences its own abilities and skills simply as a restoration of what belongs to nature. And that is why medicine represents a peculiar unity of theoretical knowledge and practical know-how within the domain of the modern sciences.

By applying her personal and experiential knowing how and knowing that, the expert nurse is able to make informed clinical judgements rather than merely responding according to the dictates of research findings. Whereas the research-based nurse is working to a formula or algorithm which states, for example, that in situation S, research tells us that we should make the response R; the expert makes an informed judgement of the situation which takes the findings of research into account, but which also draws on her accumulation of experience and her knowledge of the individual patient, and indeed of herself. In the following chapter, we shall explore how those judgements can be made.

Notes to Chapter 1

1. The Church, however, did not feel the same compulsion. Galileo was heavily persecuted for advocating what was seen in the early seventeenth century as a heretical theory, and it was only in 1992 that Pope John Paul II formally (and rather belatedly) apologized to Galileo on behalf of the Church.

REFLECTIVE BREAK

EXPLORING MY OWN KNOWLEDGE

Now turn back to the table which you started to fill in for the Reflective Break on page 26. From Table 1.2 categorize the kinds of knowledge that you identified in column 1. Write them in the empty column 4. For example, if you identified that you know how to perform a dressing according to the procedures manual, you would categorize that as scientific practical knowledge.

Now think about and write down your answers to the following questions:

What kinds of knowledge did you identify?

Which was the most common?

Were there any that you did not identify? If so, which?

Which kinds of knowledge were you most confident about?

What does that tell you about how you make clinical decisions? In particular, to what extent do you rely on professional judgement?

2. The opposite effect, known as a type I error, occurs when a statistically significant rise on, say a depression rating, does not produce a clinically significant lifting of depression.
3. The generalizing of experiential knowledge to new situations is not the same as the process of statistical generalizability discussed earlier. In order to avoid confusion, other writers have used the term 'transferability' (Guba and Lincoln, 1989) or 'fittingness' (Sandelowski, 1986; Koch, 1994) to refer to the generalization from one case to another. This form of generalizability will be discussed in more detail in Part Two of the book.
4. World 1, incidentally, is the world of physical objects, and has no knowledge-base associated with it.

2

Professional judgement

Developing personal theory

The paradigm of technical rationality maintains that nursing practice should be research based, that the findings from scientific research should be employed to generate theories which are then implemented by practitioners. We have seen, however, that there are technical and ethical limitations to the application of scientific research to nursing practice situations, and that the blind and rigid adherence to the technical rationality paradigm produces what Benner referred to as novice nurses and creates a gap between theory and practice. What is required is 'an epistemology of practice which places technical problem solving within a broader context of reflective enquiry' (Schön, 1983). In the previous chapter, I argued along with Clarke *et al.* that the nurse's own professional judgement, consisting of a combination of personal and experiential knowledge in addition to the knowledge obtained from scientific research, is just such an epistemology of practice, and that Benner was also advocating the use of a form of professional judgement when she wrote about intuitive grasp and expertise.

In the past, nursing has taken professional judgement for granted, assuming that it just develops with time, and has not given a great deal of thought to what it is, where it comes from, or how it can be developed. Thus, although Benner had a huge influence in popularizing the notion of expertise, arguing that nurses should, and often do, base their clinical decisions on professional judgement rather than on scientific research findings, she did not have much to say about what this professional judgement or expertise is, and argued, in fact, that we can probably never know.

Our next task, then, is to extend Benner's work and explore the nature of professional judgement by examining how the various types of nursing knowledge might combine not only to generate theory, but also to inform practice. Having established what professional judgement is, we will then be in a position to develop systematic, informed, publicly accountable ways of arriving at it in the same way that the scientific research process generates scientific knowledge.

Reflective practice

We will start our exploration of professional judgement with the concept of reflective practice. Partly due to Benner's work, reflection is now widely accepted as an important part of the nurse's repertoire of skills, and has been defined as:

> the retrospective contemplation of practice undertaken in order to uncover the knowledge used in a particular situation, by analyzing and interpreting the information recalled. The reflective practitioner may speculate how the situation might have been handled differently and what other knowledge would have been helpful.
>
> (Fitzgerald, 1994)

The important point to note is that reflective practice is retrospective and takes place after, and usually away from, the clinical situation which is being reflected on. Schön (1983) referred to this 'retrospective contemplation of practice' as reflection-on-action, which results in what Boyd and Fales (1983) claimed to be a 'changed conceptual perspective'. By altering the conceptual perspective of the nurse, the process of reflection-on-action turns clinical experience into personal and experiential knowledge.[1] It is largely irrelevant how much experience a nurse has; if she does not reflect and learn from that experience it will never help her to improve her practice. Indeed, I am sure that most of us can think of nurses with twenty or more years of experience whose practice is no better (and is often worse!) than it was twenty years ago.

Clearly, then, there is more to being an expert practitioner than possessing twenty years' experience; that experience must be processed and turned into experiential or personal knowledge before it can be used, just as the data which we obtain from scientific research have to be processed and integrated into our existing body of scientific knowledge. By reflecting on our actions, in clinical supervision or through diary keeping, we are able to examine our personal nursing experiences and attempt to make sense of them in the same way that a researcher examines, orders and structures her data.

But reflection-on-action is more than simply recounting past experiences: it is an active learning process. As Andrews (1996) pointed out:

> Reflection is, therefore, not to be confused with thinking about practice, which may only involve recalling what has occurred rather than learning from it.

Reflection-on-action is a method of learning which results in personal knowledge about the situation being reflected on.

Personal knowledge, then, is processed experience, and experiential knowledge is clusters of these processed experiences, the sum of all my personal knowledge about a particular situation. Thus, in situation S:

EXPERIENCE OF S + REFLECTION = PERSONAL
KNOWLEDGE OF S
Σ (sum) PERSONAL KNOWLEDGE OF S = EXPERIENTIAL
KNOWLEDGE OF S

Schön also identified a second type of reflective practice which he called reflection-*in*-action. This involves working with the personal and experiential knowledge that results from reflection-*on*-action in real time in the practice setting. It entails developing a theory about the clinical situation that the nurse finds herself in, what Schön (1983) referred to as 'a new theory of the unique case', testing out that theory in practice, and modifying it accordingly. Because reflection-in-action generates and tests theories, Schön also referred to it as on-the-spot experimenting, and saw it as a form of research. Thus:

> When the practitioner reflects in action in a case he perceives as unique, paying attention to phenomena and surfacing his intuitive under-standing of them, his experience is at once exploratory, move testing, and hypothesis testing. The three functions are fulfilled by the very same actions. And from this fact follows the distinctive character of experimenting in practice.
>
> (Schön, 1987)

As we shall see later, Schön's notion of reflection-in-action as hypothesis testing is particularly pertinent to expert practice.

Personal theory

Clarke *et al.* (1996) referred to the kind of theory created through reflection-in-action as 'nursing theory', and claimed that it:

provides the rationale appropriate for practice at the moment of acting in a particular context. When nurses reflect in action, they draw on their theories about nursing to generate the knowing in action.

It is this theorizing, or reflecting on what might happen, that Van Manen (1991) referred to as anticipative reflection.

However, the kind of theory produced as part of reflection-in-action is very different from the theory produced by scientific research. Just as a scientific theory gives order to scientific knowledge so that we can use it to describe, explain and make predictions about the world, so reflection-in-action generates a form of theory that structures personal and experiential knowledge, an *experiential* theory of practice rather than a scientific one, a theory which attempts to *explain* and *predict* what we do in clinical settings rather than merely informing and directing practice.

Carr and Kemmis have attempted to describe this kind of theory in the discipline of education. They argued that as well as traditional scientific theory which refers to 'the products of theoretical enquiries like psychology or sociology ... presented in the form of general laws, causal explanations, and the like' (Carr and Kemmis, 1986), there is also a type of theory emerging from, and embedded in, our own personal practice:

> A "practice", then, is not some kind of thoughtless behaviour which exists separately from "theory" and to which theory can be "applied". Furthermore, all practices, like all observations, have "theory" embedded in them.
>
> (Carr and Kemmis, 1986)

Schön (1987) referred to these personal, practice-based theories as theories-in-use, 'implicit in our patterns of spontaneous behaviour', while Usher and Bryant coined the term 'informal theory', and added:

> Since without such a "theory" practice would be random and purposeless, we can say that it "forms" practice. It enables practitioners to make sense of what they are doing and thus appears to have an *enabling* function.
>
> (Usher and Bryant, 1989)

I will use the term 'personal theory' for this theory of practice,[2] since this kind of theory is not generalizable in the way that scientific theory is, but is personal to the practitioner and specific to the situation it is derived from. Personal theory, then, is conceptually linked to practice; indeed, it forms part of the definition of practice, since without personal theory, practice degenerates into random, purpose-less behaviour. Personal theory is theory-in-use, theory *in* practice rather than *of* practice, and whereas personal knowledge can be constructed during the process of reflection-*on*-action, away from the practice setting in which the experiences it is based on were gathered, personal theory-building can only happen through reflection-*in*-action, in and during practice.

Personal theory is only of relevance to us if, ultimately, it results in better nursing practice. We have seen that scientific theory is very useful for generating new scientific knowledge, but not so good for making predictions about individual practice situations. Personal theory, on the other hand, tells us little about generalizable scientific knowledge, but can be very useful in helping us to respond to unique individual patients in unique individual settings. When I encounter a new practice situation, I can summon my personal and experiential knowledge and transform it into a theoretical explana-tion of the problem I am faced with. This personal theory, a theory relating to a specific clinical decision in a specific situation, can then be tested in that very situation, and accepted, modified or discarded in favour of a better theory. The point is, however, that I have not only constructed a new theory about my practice, but that in the process of doing so, I have brought about real and meaningful therapeutic interventions.

Thus, unlike traditional scientific theory, which can be (and often is) constructed without going anywhere near a practice setting, and which is then applied *to* practice, personal theory about my nursing practice can only be generated through being a nurse, and arises *from* practice. This is an important distinction, since personal theory cannot be constructed by academics and researchers who are not also practitioners; personal theory is generated and owned by *nurses*. But the real strength of personal theory-building is that it offers a process by which nurses can make rational clinical decisions in the practice setting. By theorizing on the possible reasons for, and events leading up to, a clinical situation, we can make informed, conscious decisions about how to act in that situation.

The educationalist John Dewey, who did much to popularize experiential learning in the early years of the twentieth century, used the term 'purpose' for the construction and application of personal theory, and described it as 'a plan and method of action based upon foresight of the consequences of acting under given observed conditions in a certain way' (Dewey, 1938). He claimed that it consisted of:

(1) observation of surrounding conditions; (2) knowledge of what has happened in similar situations in the past, a knowledge obtained partly by recollection and partly from the information, advice, and warning of those who have had a wider experience; and (3) judgement which puts together what is observed and what is recalled to see what they signify.

(Dewey, 1938)

We can see that Dewey's 'observation of surrounding conditions' is similar to what I have referred to as personal knowledge, that is, knowledge of the context in which the theory is being generated, including knowledge of the patient. His 'recollection of what has happened in the past' is what I have called experiential knowledge, knowledge of previous situations generated by reflection-on-action. His 'information, advice and warning of those who have had a wider experience' could be construed as scientific knowledge, generalizable knowledge which is applied to individual situations. And 'the judgement which puts together what is observed and what is recalled to see what they signify' is the personal theory itself, a combination of personal, experiential and scientific knowledge, synthesized for the purpose of understanding a particular and unique clinical problem.

But although Dewey outlined the components which go to make up a personal theory, he offered little insight into the process of the 'judgement' through which they are combined. Why, for example, do we choose *this* piece of personal knowledge rather than *that* piece? Why one particular previous experience rather than another? Why the findings from study A and not from study B? And how are they to be combined? Should we give more weight to this piece of personal knowledge or that piece of experiential knowledge? Is it even possible to divide knowledge into pieces in this way?

The logic of personal theory

One possible answer to these questions comes from the branch of computer science known as artificial intelligence and, in particular, from the study of so-called 'expert systems'. Expert systems are computer programs which attempt to mimic or explain the behaviour and decision-making processes of human experts; for example, chess-playing computers (although in this case, there is no attempt to mimic the decision-making of chess Grand Masters, only the resulting behaviour). There is a certain irony in this approach to the study of theory-building in nursing, since it was Hubert Dreyfus' rejection of expert systems as an explanation for human expertise that led Benner to her conclusions about the role of intuition in nursing.

Dreyfus (1979) argued that the linear, algorithmic, 'if-then' chains of reasoning by which expert systems are programmed were totally inadequate as an explanation of the way that real people make decisions in real situations, and concluded that human expert decision-making was an intuitive and, if not an irrational, then certainly an *a*rational process. Thus, in describing the way that doctors theorize and make decisions, Dreyfus and Dreyfus (1986) claimed:

> In reality, a patient is viewed by the experienced doctor as a unique case and treated on the basis of intuitively perceived similarity with situations previously encountered. That kind of wisdom, unfortunately, cannot be shared and thereby made the basis of a doctor's rational decision.

Recent developments in computer expert systems seem to suggest, however, that this kind of wisdom can not only be shared, but that it can be modelled and understood in a rational way.

The breakthrough in our understanding of the way in which experts theorize and make decisions came about following the development of a new branch of computer programming known as fuzzy logic (Kosko, 1994). Fuzzy logic does not rely on the traditional *serial* approach to computer expert systems of on-off, if-then, either-or decision making, but on a *parallel* approach which not only processes all the available information at the same time, but assigns each piece a 'fuzzy', analogue value such as 'quite important' or 'not terribly relevant' in much the same way that people categorize their knowledge. This enables the computer to assign a 'fuzzy weighted average' to a particular decision, based on a consideration of the relative importance of a wide range of different items of knowledge and information. Kosko argued that human experts function in a very similar way. Here, he described how an expert judge comes to a decision:

> The judge weighs up the principles and cites case precedents to back up the weights. The judge does not give the weights as numbers... but they are a matter of degree. Some weights rank more important than others. Some judges know more law and see more connections and cite more cases than others do. The judge cites these cases to justify her ruling. She does not point out an audit trail in a rule book. She gives what looks a lot like a fuzzy weighted average.
>
> (Kosko, 1994)

And so it is with nurses. The expert nurse weighs up her personal knowledge of the patient she is working with, she considers past cases, she draws on relevant theory and research, and she arrives at a synthesis, a fuzzy weighted average which assigns different degrees of importance and relevance to the different pieces of knowledge which make up the personal theory which informs her decision. And like Kosko's judge, she does not give numerical values to these pieces of knowledge, she leaves no audit trail.

Kosko went as far as to claim that fuzzy logic is no logic at all, and that:

> we have only one decision rule: *I'll do it if it feels right.* The formal logic we learnt in tenth-grade geometry class has little to do with it.
>
> (Kosko, 1994)

Kosko was right to assert that formal propositional logic has nothing to do with fuzzy decision-making, but wrong in his conclusion that fuzzy decisions are based merely on what feels right at the time. In fact, Kosko's fuzzy judge is employing a little-known form of inductive reasoning known as abduction or what Harman (1965) referred to as 'inference to the best explanation'.

Abduction was first proposed by the philosopher C.S. Peirce, and has been described as:

> a form of inference that goes from data describing something to a hypothesis that best explains or accounts for the data. Thus abduction is a kind of theory-forming or interpretive inference.
>
> (Josephson and Josephson, 1994)

Josephson and Josephson used an example from *Winnie-the-Pooh* (Milne, 1926) to illustrate abductive reasoning:

> It had HUNNY written on it, but, just to make sure, he took off the paper cover and looked at it, and it *looked* just like honey. "But you can never tell", said Pooh. "I remember my uncle saying once that he had seen cheese just this colour". So he put his tongue in, and took a large lick.

Pooh wanted to know what was in the jar, and he had two pieces of data to help him decide. First, the jar had HUNNY written on it, and secondly, the substance in the jar looked just like honey. However, cheese had also been observed to look similar to the substance in the jar. There are thus two competing theories: the substance is cheese or the substance is honey. Clearly, the latter theory best accounts for the data (after all, the label does say HUNNY), and Pooh tested this out by taking a lick.

Josephson and Josephson argued that abductive reasoning is employed by people as well as bears, and pointed out instances in all walks of life, including science, history and literature.[3] Kosko's fuzzy judge is employing abduction: she infers a theory that best explains the accumulation of evidence, and uses this theory to formulate a ruling on the case. Similarly, the expert nurse employs the logic of abduction to construct a personal theory based on the relevant personal, experiential and scientific knowledge of the case.

Abduction is a form of inductive reasoning, and we have already seen that induction can never result in certainty; it merely provides the theory that best fits the available data (that is why Pooh had to confirm his theory with a lick).

Abductions are therefore based on probability, but we have already seen that the traditional theory of statistical probability tells us nothing about individual clinical decisions.

Josephson and Josephson (1994) acknowledged this, claiming that 'in practice it seems that rough qualitative confidence levels on the hypotheses are enough to support abductions'. The philosopher Rudolf Carnap described this qualitative form of probability as inductive probability, which is 'ascribed to a hypothesis with respect to a body of evidence' (Carnap, 1970). He continued:

> In most cases in ordinary discourse, even among scientists, inductive probability is not specified by a numerical value but merely as being high or low or, in a comparative judgement, as being higher than another probability.

Thus, when a bookmaker fixes the odds against a particular horse winning the Grand National at five to one, she is giving a statistical probability of one chance in six that it will win. However, when you or I say that it is highly probable that the horse will win, we are stating an inductive probability based on Josephson and Josephson's 'rough qualitative confidence levels'.

Furthermore, in making such a judgement, we are using the logic of abduction, employing our 'research-based' knowledge of the horse's previous form, our experiential knowledge of how similar horses have fared in similar situations, and our personal knowledge of the sort of conditions that this horse favours.

There is clearly a very close relationship between Kosko's fuzzy logic, Peirce's abduction and Carnap's inductive probability, and all three underpin the decision-making process of the expert. As Carnap pointed out, these 'fuzzy' judgements are based on the totality of relevant evidence available to the person making the decision. Like Kosko, Carnap used a legal example in his explanation of inductive probability which bears a striking resemblance to the way in which Kosko's fuzzy judge came to her decision:

> If a member of a jury says that the defendant is very probably innocent
> or that, of two witnesses A and B who have made contradictory
> statements, it is more probable that A lied than that B did, he means it
> with respect to the evidence that was presented in the trial plus any
> psychological or other relevant knowledge of a general nature he may
> possess.
>
> (Carnap, 1970)

The juror is weighing up the evidence in relation to her personal,
experiential and scientific knowledge of the case, and deciding,
through the logic of abduction, on the inductive probability that the
defendant is innocent.

The expert nurse, I would argue, works in a similar way, and therefore follows a logical process in constructing her personal theory,
albeit a fuzzy logical process. When she formulates the personal
theory that it is highly probable that Mr Brown would wish to be
told that he is dying, her judgement is not based on the statistical
probability of empirical scientific research, that is, on what *most*
patients would wish, nor is it based on some mystical, unknowable
intuition, but on an inductive probability arrived at by weighing up all
the available personal, experiential and scientific knowledge through
the process of abductive reasoning.

Personal theory and professional judgement

Expertise, praxis and professional judgement

But this is only half the story. Having formulated a personal theory
which accounts for the clinical problem she is faced with, the nurse
must now transform that theory into action. We should remember,
however, that a theory (and that includes a personal theory) is provi-
sional, it is our 'best guess' or 'inference to the best explanation' about
the uncertain situation that we find ourselves in, and as such, it must
be tested. Fortunately, one of the features of a personal theory is that
it is formulated by a practitioner actually in a practice situation, and
so the act of testing the theory is also the act of applying it. As Schön
(1983) pointed out:

> The practitioner allows himself to experience surprise, puzzlement, or
> confusion in a situation which he finds uncertain or unique. He reflects
> on the phenomena before him, and on the prior understandings which
> have been implicit in his behavior. He carries out an experiment *which
> serves to generate both a new understanding of the phenomena and a
> change in the situation* (my emphasis).

In testing a personal theory, the nurse is therefore also making a clinical intervention. She is formulating a hypothesis, based on her theory, of the probable clinical outcomes of certain actions, she is acting in accordance with that hypothesis, and she is assessing whether the predicted outcomes have occurred. And as Elstein and Bordage (1988) have pointed out, 'it seems practically impossible to reason without hypotheses whenever the data base is as complex as it typically is in clinical problems'.

Returning to the example of Pooh, he employed abductive reasoning to formulate the personal theory that the jar contained honey, he generated the hypothesis, based on his theory, that the substance in the jar, if licked, would taste like honey, and he tested his hypothesis by taking a lick. He then assessed whether the predicted outcome had occurred: ' "Yes", he said, "it is. No doubt about that" '.

Stenhouse (1984a) described this process of theory-building and hypothesis testing in terms of prudence and perceptiveness. Prudence is defined in the *Oxford English Dictionary* as 'the ability to discern the most suitable, politic or profitable course of action; practical wisdom, discretion'. It is clearly related to Harman's 'inference to the best explanation', and culminates in the formation of a personal theory about how to respond to a specific clinical situation. Perceptiveness is 'the capacity to interpret situations rapidly and at depth and to revise interpretations in the light of experience' (Stenhouse, 1984a), and is the result of testing and modifying that personal theory. This cyclical process, in which personal theories are continuously formulated, tested, modified, retested, and so on, is shown in Figure 2.1.

Clarke *et al.* (1996) have more recently referred to this process of theory generation and testing as 'deliberative reflection', and claimed that it requires practitioners:

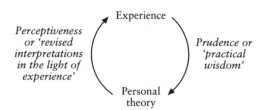

Figure 2.1 *Prudence, perceptiveness and professional judgement (after Stenhouse, 1984a).*

to draw on both their knowledge of the context in which they are working and their non-contextualized professional knowledge ... [i]n order to make decisions about appropriate courses of action and to solve the myriad of problems that confront them in their professional work.

I have previously described this process of theory generation and testing as 'praxis', the coming together of theory and practice as a unified whole (Rolfe, 1993, 1996). Van Manen (1990) used the same term, stating that 'by praxis we mean thoughtful action: action full of thought and thought full of action', whereas McNiff *et al.* (1996) defined it as 'informed, committed action that gives rise to knowledge rather than just successful action'. I believe that it is also the very process that Benner's expert nurse is engaging in, albeit unconsciously, when she is displaying an intuitive grasp of a clinical situation.

Benner defined intuition as 'understanding without a rationale' (Benner and Tanner, 1987), and claimed that it is an unconscious process whereby the practitioner is largely unaware of how and where her practice knowledge comes from; she just seems to know the right thing to do at the right time. She cited an expert psychiatric nurse to illustrate this point:

> When I say to a doctor "the patient is psychotic", I don't always know how to legitimize the statement. But I am never wrong. Because I know psychosis from inside out. And I feel that, and I know it, and I trust it.
> (Benner, 1984)

Intuitive grasp is not only an unconscious process, but according to Benner, it is also unknowable. The nurse practising at this level is, she claimed, not following rules and 'this multifaceted knowledge ... cannot readily be put into abstract principles or even explicit guidelines'. Furthermore, 'if experts are made to attend to the particulars or to a formal model or rule, their performance actually deteriorates' (Benner, 1984).

Although widely accepted by the nursing profession, this view of expertise is not without its critics. The most common objection is that Benner's model of expertise as unknowable intuitive grasp leads to a form of elitism in which self-styled experts need not justify their practice to the 'lower orders' of nurses. Like Benner's psychiatric nurse, the expert is never wrong, and because her expertise is unfathomable, it is also safe from attack; she does not have to justify her decisions because she *cannot* justify her decisions. She just knows that she is always right. Schön (1983) perfectly summed up this objection (albeit before Benner had even published her book) when he wrote:

When people use terms such as "art" and "intuition", they usually intend to terminate discussion rather than to open up inquiry. It is as though the practitioner says to his academic colleague, "While I do not accept *your* view of knowledge, I cannot describe my own." Sometimes, indeed, the practitioner appears to say, "My kind of knowledge is indescribable," or even, "I will not attempt to describe it lest I paralyse myself." These attitudes have contributed to a widening rift between the universities and the professions, research and practice, thought and action.

Thus, in contrast to Benner's view, many psychologists and philosophers have argued that this sort of intuition *is* a rational, rule-bound process, albeit an unconscious one. In fact, Benner (1984) at one point stated the logical process underlying intuitive grasp quite explicitly, pointing out that 'expertise develops when the clinician tests and refines propositions, hypotheses, and principle-based expectations in actual practice situations'. Andrews (1996) supported this view when she claimed that 'intuition may, therefore, be viewed as a complex critical skill that is the result of modification of personal theory through reflecting in action'.

It is possible, then, that Benner's expert nurse is unconsciously solving clinical problems in a structured and logical way by formulating and testing hypotheses derived from personal theories, although she is unaware that she is doing so. The difference between my model of praxis and Benner's concept of expertise is therefore that the former is conscious whereas the latter is unconscious. To avoid confusion, I will refer in this book to the problem-solving process itself as 'professional judgement', to its conscious manifestation as 'praxis', and to its unconscious use as 'intuitive grasp' or 'expertise'.

However, the contrast between praxis and expertise is far more dramatic than the difference between a conscious and an unconscious decision-making process would seem to suggest, and by being aware of the process of professional judgement, the practitioner *transcends* expertise and moves to a higher level of practice, beyond Benner's stage of expert.

The most important difference between unconscious expertise as Benner described it, and conscious praxis, is that whereas the expert acts smoothly, quickly and unconsciously, almost at spinal cord level, and is unable to verbalize why she responded in the way that she did, praxis requires a particular sort of mindfulness which involves an intense and conscious concentration on the task at hand.

Also, whereas the expert is a *reflective* practitioner, whose practice is based on experiential know-how acquired through reflection-on-action away from the clinical setting and after the event, praxis is concerned with reflection-in-action, with on-the-spot experimenting and with the generation of knowledge and theory in the practice situation during practice itself; that is, with *reflexive* practice. I am not claiming that the expert nurse does not engage in the process of professional judgement, only that she is not aware that she is doing so, and that this lack of awareness is a limiting factor on her practice.

The importance of self-awareness is highlighted in the distinction made by Stenhouse (1977) between informal and formal practice. The informal practitioner relies on her intuition, sensitivity and charisma, and cannot or will not verbalize her *modus operandi*. Formal practice, on the other hand, is based on the assumption that practice can be developed experimentally as an art. The formal practitioner is constantly seeking to improve her practice, whereas informal practice leaves no room for experiment or for a formal and structured route to improvement.

Thus, because the reflective expert practitioner is unable to verbalize how she arrives at her clinical decisions, she is unable consciously to improve her clinical decision-making process in the light of her past experiences. In the case of the psychiatric nurse described earlier, how is she to develop her diagnostic skills when she is unaware of how she makes her diagnoses? All she can do is continue accumulating paradigm cases in the hope that they will somehow transform into expert practice. Or perhaps Benner would argue that the expert nurse has no need to improve since, by her own admission, she is never wrong. But such an attitude leads not only to complacency but to burn-out. The nurse who believes she has achieved perfection has nowhere further to go and her practice soon becomes stagnant.

The reflexive nurse–practitioner, on the other hand, is fully aware of the process by which she makes care decisions. Furthermore, because praxis is a conscious process, she is able to modify the care she gives in direct and immediate response to its effects. Thus, not only is clinical change brought about by her actions, but refinements to her practice occur in response to that clinical change in a continuous feedback loop. Because she is conscious of the way in which she integrates personal, scientific and experiential knowledge into her practice, she is also able to modify that practice in direct and immediate response to changes in her knowledge-base, and reflexive practice is therefore in a continuous state of development.

A model of professional judgement

It can be seen from Figure 2.2 that professional judgements integrate personal, experiential and scientific knowledge, reflection-on-action, reflection-in-action and personal theory in a process that both generates further knowledge and brings about changes to practice through the formulation and testing of personal theories.

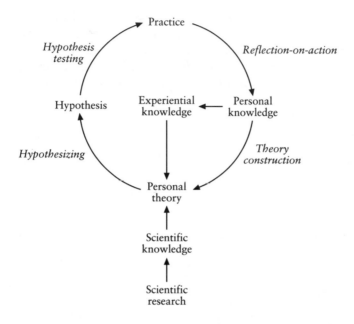

Figure 2.2   *A model of professional judgement.*

The concept of professional judgement should be of great importance and relevance to all practising nurses. It is a framework for articulating and justifying the experiential and personal knowledge which raises the status of the nurse from a mere technician and doctor's assistant to a fully autonomous professional, able to make clinical decisions without recourse to procedures and guidelines. Furthermore, it transforms her from the implementor of other people's theories into the generator and tester of her own knowledge and theory. It is important to recognize, then, that a professional judgement does not end with the formulation of a theory about the best course of action to take in a given situation, but that it tests out the theory in practice and is modified according to the outcomes of that testing. Professional judgements are therefore not static in the way that judgements based on scientific knowledge are, but are dynamic, organic, growing judgements which develop as a result of our experiences.

It should be borne in mind that this model of professional judgement did not arise from scientific research, but from my experiences of being a nurse and a teacher and my reflections on those experiences, as well as vicariously from the experiences of others. It therefore does not constitute scientific knowledge but experiential theoretical knowledge based on clusters of paradigm cases. Furthermore, this particular experiential knowledge has made the transition from world 2, the world of thoughts and ideas, to world 3, the world of the contents of books and libraries, by being written down and published.

It can be seen from Figure 2.2 that professional judgements begin with the process of reflection-on-action, the transformation of practice-based experiences into personal knowledge. This reflection-on-action can happen in a number of ways: in clinical supervision, by keeping a reflective diary, through formal critical incident analysis, or simply by sitting down and reflecting on experiences. The personal knowledge which results from the process can then be taken back into the clinical setting in order to rectify immediately an existing problem, or else it can be stored away as part of the practitioner's repertoire of paradigm cases and employed to construct experiential knowledge.

This personal and experiential knowledge can also be used to generate personal theory through the process of reflection-*in*-action. When confronted with a problem, such as the earlier example of a terminally ill patient who asks whether he is dying, the nurse employing professional judgement draws primarily on the body of personal knowledge she has built up about that particular patient in order to reach a decision on how to respond.

However, that personal knowledge will be supported from the nurse's repertoire of experiential knowledge in the form of paradigm cases, which might contain similar instances, and from her body of scientific, research-based knowledge and theory. Thus, as well as knowledge about the patient concerned, she might also draw on previous situations when she either gave or did not give the requested information, knowledge of the ethical implications of giving the information, the findings from scientific research studies, and psychological theories of counselling.

By combining and synthesizing these very different forms of knowledge into a 'fuzzy weighted average' based on the logic of abduction and inductive probability, she is able to construct a personal theory about *this* patient in *this* situation by reflecting-in-action. Her personal theory might be, for example, that this patient genuinely wishes to know whether he is dying in order to put his affairs in order, and that he is psychologically equipped to deal with the consequences of being told.

Because personal theory is constructed *in* practice, actually in the clinical situation in direct response to a problem, it can be immediately applied by forming a hypothesis based on the theory and testing out predictions derived from it in the practice setting. If the predicted outcomes occur, then not only is the theory upheld, but a clinical intervention based on that theory has been implemented. If, on the other hand, the predicted outcomes do not occur, then the modified clinical situation is reassessed, and a new theory is generated. In the words of Gadamer (1996) 'every mistake revenges itself and ... a permanent process of learning and self-correction is sustained through the experience of success or the lack of it'.

The hypothesis in the above example might be that if the information that the patient is dying is given in a sensitive, supportive and caring manner, his anxiety and distress will reduce. This prediction is tested by telling the patient, and having made her intervention, the nurse continues around the cycle again by making a new assessment of the transformed situation, that is, whether or not the patient's anxiety has reduced, generating further experiential knowledge, and so on.

Thus, theory and practice are brought together as two parts of an indivisible whole. Personal theory is generated in response to a specific clinical situation by combining personal knowledge relating to that situation, experiential knowledge in the form of paradigm cases and generalizable scientific knowledge and theory through reflection-in-action, and brings about change in the clinical situation as a result of being tested. Of course, there is always the possibility that the hypothesized outcomes do not occur, that the patient's anxiety level does not reduce, and in that case the theory would need to be modified, or a new personal theory would need to be constructed. However, the probability of a personal theory successfully translating into practice is far greater than that of a scientific theory, simply because extra personal and experiential knowledge is brought to bear on the clinical problem. The gap between theory and practice is therefore very much reduced.

REFLECTIVE BREAK

USING THE MODEL OF PROFESSIONAL JUDGEMENT

Think of a clinical situation you have been a part of with a patient you know well, in which you made a nursing decision to respond in a particular way. If you cannot identify one, think of a clinical decision you might be faced with in the future which involves a patient you know well.

Try to identify the personal theory that your decision was based on.

What personal knowledge did you employ in constructing the theory?

Did you have any experiential knowledge in the form of paradigm cases – things that worked or did not work in similar situations in the past?

What scientific knowledge informed your decision?

How did you test out your theory? How did you verify your hypothesis?

Did you need to modify your theory in the light of your findings?

There are clear parallels between scientific theory construction and professional judgement. Both generate knowledge through a systematic process of enquiry: formal research in the case of science, and reflection-on-action in the case of professional judgement. Both structure that knowledge in the form of scientific or personal theory, and both employ that theory to generate new knowledge and to bring about changes in practice.

It should be noted, however, that in many ways the personal theory which results from professional judgement is very different from scientific theory. Personal theory is context-specific, referring only to *this* patient (or this jar of honey) in *this* situation, and exists only in relation to practice, arising out of a specific practice setting and consequently informing our actions in that particular setting. Scientific theory, on the other hand, refers to global, generalizable situations and exists independently of practice. Furthermore, although the process of making professional judgements has been presented in a linear, logical way, it should not be confused with the logic of positivist science. As Clarke *et al.* (1996) pointed out:

> The process of arriving at a professional judgement in this way may appear to be grounded in a positivist form of logic, but the nature of the form of knowledge on which the practitioner draws means that it cannot be truly positivist in nature. The knowledge of the practitioner is grounded in interpretive judgements of a dialectical form, constructed by the reflections of the practitioner, rather than in "facts" that can be externally verified. The process may appear positivist because in the practical life of the professional, the true complexity must go unnoticed, so that the action and communication can be managed.

In fact, there are a number of differences between scientific and personal theory, which are summarized in Table 2.1. In particular, personal theory is specific to a particular clinical situation and has no application outside of that situation. Unlike scientific theories, which, if well constructed, tend to be fairly robust and long-lasting, personal theories are ephemeral, and new theories are required for each new clinical situation the nurse finds herself in.

Personal theories, then, are constantly being generated, tested, modified and discarded in what Stenhouse (1985a) referred to as laboratory experiments. He continued (and remember, he was writing about education rather than nursing):

> There is thus a need for the development of educational laboratories. In them we shall have to control conditions so that we can simulate faith-

Table 2.1 The differences between scientific and personal theory

Scientific theory	Personal theory
Organizes and makes sense of what we already know about the world in general	Organizes and makes sense of what we already know about specific individual people or situations
Can be used to make predictions about what will happen in the world in general	Can be used to make predictions about what will happen to specific people in specific situations
Is generated by researchers and academics as part of the formal research process	Is generated by practitioners as part of their everyday practice
Is based on formal logic and statistical probability	Is based on fuzzy logic and inductive probability
Is generalizable to other people and other situations	Is personal and specific to this situation, and cannot be generalized to other people, or even to the same person in other situations
Can be generated away from the practice setting without going anywhere near a clinical area	Can only be generated in practice settings
Is totally separate from practice, but can be employed to direct practice	Is generated *from* practice, is immediately applied back *into* practice, and cannot be separated from practice

fully those of real classrooms ... But wait a minute! That would seem to imply that wherever there is a real classroom there is a potential educational laboratory. Just so. The best designed educational laboratories are in the charge of teachers, not of researchers.

The implications for nursing are obvious. To paraphrase Stenhouse, wherever there is a real clinical area there is a potential nursing laboratory, and the best designed nursing laboratories are in the charge of nurses, not of researchers.

Clearly, then, by raising the status and importance of personal theory, we also raise the status and importance of the practising nurse from the applier of other people's theories to the generator and tester of her own theories. I have referred elsewhere to these different kinds of nurses, the theory applier and the theory generator, as the nurse-technician and the nurse–practitioner (Rolfe, 1996).

Theory, practice and the nurse–practitioner

We have seen that personal theory is the vital, dynamic component of professional judgement which serves to integrate personal, experiential and scientific knowledge through the process of abduction. It not only enables us to make sense of the relationship between these different kinds of knowledge and demonstrates that all three types are important for effective practice, but more importantly, it also helps bring about changes to practice through reflection-in-action or on-the-spot experimenting. Personal theory and practice cannot therefore be separated, and there is clearly a close relationship between the knowledge-base of a nurse and the way in which she practises, which will now be explored further.

When she first enters the profession, the nurse is at a 'pre-novice' stage, and will have little or no scientific knowledge related to nursing and no experiential knowledge of past cases. She will not, however, be entirely useless (although she might well not be particularly safe either), since she will probably bring with her a degree of innate or learned ability in relating to people and building therapeutic relationships. The psychotherapist Carl Rogers (1974) believed that this innate ability takes the form of deeply held 'therapeutic attitudes' which we draw on in interpersonal situations, and which facilitate psychological healing.

The beginning nurse who is able to form interpersonal relationships will also quickly build a body of personal knowledge about her individual patients, knowledge about their personal history, their likes and dislikes, and to some extent, their medical and nursing problems. Thus, personal knowledge is usually the first to develop, although at this level much of it is not consciously acknowledged by the nurse and is informally structured.

As her formal education proceeds, the nurse will begin to develop a body of scientific knowledge from the disciplines of biology, psychology and sociology, as well as from nurse theorists and researchers. Ideally, this scientific knowledge should complement her personal knowledge, but there is some evidence, not just from nursing but from all the caring professions that, in fact, it overwhelms and suppresses it. It would appear that many nurses at this level, which is comparable to Benner's novice stage, tend to reject the personal knowledge and innate attitudes of the beginner in favour of a reliance on scientific knowledge to inform their clinical practice, and part of the reason for this trend must rest with the relatively low status given to the former types of knowledge in nursing and with the increasing importance attached to a scientific research base for nursing practice.

As the nurse continues to gain experience, the individual paradigm cases which make up her personal knowledge begin to cluster around different patient-care issues to form an experiential knowledge-base. This marks the beginning of professional judgement, and at this level, the nurse often gets her first personal taste of the theory–practice gap, that is, the dissonance created by the alternative courses of action prescribed by her experiential knowledge and her scientific knowledge.

It is no longer easy for her to deny the value of her personal and experiential knowledge, and many nurses at this level begin to realize that practice based entirely on scientific knowledge and research does not always produce the optimum care for each individual patient, and that sometimes the best care comes from deliberately flouting research-based practice. Recall, for example, MacGuire's observation, quoted earlier, that 'research, for a variety of reasons, has not always addressed the concerns of clinical nurses and frequently does not produce the kind of reliable guide to practice that practitioners require'.

As the nurse begins to acquire personal and experiential knowledge, she is therefore faced with a dilemma: whether to continue to practice as a technician, applying generalizable scientific knowledge to the unique and individual practice situations she finds herself in, or whether to become a nurse–practitioner and allow her professional judgement to override research-based practice.

However, the nurse who, to a greater or lesser extent, attempts to base her practice on her professional judgement and experience rather than on scientific knowledge is at a great disadvantage since she has no body of formal research on which to justify her clinical decisions. She therefore faces criticism from her nurse–technician colleagues for practising according to her own subjective whim or 'gut feeling' rather than from the perceived certainty of the technical rationality paradigm. Now look at the Reflective Break on page 62.

The problem is that the personal and experiential knowledge on which professional judgements are made is usually generated in a very *ad hoc* fashion, and a great deal of valuable experience is either not

REFLECTIVE BREAK

PROFFESIONAL JUDGEMENT AND RESEARCH-BASED KNOWLEDGE

Think of a situation where there has been a conflict between your professional judgement and the course of action prescribed by research. Write it down below.

Which course of action did you choose?

How did you justify your choice to yourself?

How did you or could you justify your choice to others?

In retrospect, would you have responded to the situation differently?

recognized or else is quickly forgotten. Furthermore, personal and experiential knowledge is not acknowledged by many academics and practitioners as a valid foundation for practice in the way that scientific knowledge is. If nurses are ever to become more than highly skilled doctors' assistants, it is necessary to expand the scope of nursing research to include the formal generation of personal knowledge and theory as well as scientific knowledge and theory. This new form of research will inevitably come into conflict with the traditional scientific research paradigm of technical rationality, one of the aims of which is to produce generalizable knowledge, knowledge which can be applied to a wide range of settings outside of the situation in which it was generated. Furthermore, whereas technical rationality tends to maintain the split between researcher and practitioner, with the former generating knowledge and theory for the latter to put into practice, personal and experiential knowledge about specific cases can only be generated by the practitioner herself.

Part of the reason for this conflict is the inability or unwillingness of the nursing profession to differentiate between clinical research and theoretical research. The traditional scientific method, and in particular, the sociological paradigm adopted by nursing, was designed to generate and test theory, and arguably one of the reasons for the current gap between theory and practice in nursing is the inability of traditional social research methods to say anything meaningful about individual practice situations.

Thus, while scientific research is appropriate and effective for generating knowledge for generalizable nursing theory, we require a new approach to the generation of the kind of knowledge and theory that is relevant to nursing practice, and as we have seen, this new approach needs to be very different from the old. What is required, then, is no less than a new paradigm; a new philosophy of what clinical research is, what it aims to do, and how it intends to do it, and the description of such a paradigm is the task of Part Two of this book.

Notes to Chapter 2

1. Clarke *et al.* (1996) claimed that reflection-on-action can look to the future as well as to the past through Van Manen's 'anticipatory reflection'. But this, I shall argue later, is not reflection-on-action as such, although it is closely related to it.

2. In a previous book and in several journal papers, I employed Usher and Bryant's term 'informal theory'. The two terms should be regarded as interchangeable.
3. Truzzi (1983) claimed that there are at least 217 cases of abductive reasoning in the Sherlock Holmes stories. Holmes, it seems, did not deduce, he abduced.

Part Two

Researching your practice

Part One of this book ended with a call for a new paradigm of clinical research carried out by practitioners themselves. However, since nursing research has modelled itself largely on the social sciences, it comes as no surprise to discover that there is little importance placed on personal and experiential nursing knowledge, and no tradition of micro clinical research carried out by practitioners with a focus on the individual patient. It is therefore to other practice-based disciplines that we have to turn, and particularly to the field of education and the work of Lawrence Stenhouse.

Stenhouse was a pioneer of practitioner research and an enthusiastic promoter of the idea that 'using research means doing research' (Stenhouse, 1981), and although he was an educationalist, most of his ideas are readily transferable to any practice-based discipline. Unfortunately, the notion of the practitioner-as-researcher has not been welcomed in nursing, where there remains a gulf between the academic researcher and the practice-based nurse. Polit and Hungler (1991) have identified the limited role that the practitioner is normally permitted to play in nursing research:

> To produce scientific research, it is necessary to develop skills in the scientific method. But it is not only nursing researchers who need to understand the scientific approach and methods of research. Nurses engaged in the practice of nursing, nursing administrators, and nursing educators all have a responsibility to identify problems that warrant scientific investigation. Professional accountability demands that nurses utilize the findings of research to perform their roles. In addition, as consumers of research, nurses are called upon to evaluate the methods used to carry out research projects to estimate the confidence that can be placed in the results.

The nurse, then, has a duty to identify problems for academic researchers to study, to evaluate the scientific credibility of those research studies, and to apply the findings to her own practice. There is no mention here of the nurse carrying out her own research, which is seen as the task of the 'nurse researcher', who is usually a practising researcher rather than a practising nurse. As Hart and Bond (1995) pointed out, this separation between researcher and practitioner

> implies to nurses that research into their own work is not something they are allowed – let alone routinely expected – to do and this in turn is likely to further entrench the practice–theory divide.

Of particular importance to this book is the notion, expressed above by Polit and Hungler, that we can estimate the credibility of the findings of a research study merely by evaluating the methods employed in that study. This was of particular concern to Stenhouse, who saw the dangers of research findings 'overriding rather than strengthening the judgement of the practitioner' (Stenhouse, 1985a). He argued that research has imposed its own agenda on practice, and that it appeals to research judgement rather than practice judgement, to the extent that we can only legitimately criticize research findings on the strength of the methodology of the study. If there are no flaws in the design and conduct of the study, then we are compelled to accept the findings as applicable to practice. Kerlinger (1964) perfectly expressed this viewpoint when he wrote:

> One cannot understand any complex human activity without some technical and methodological competence. But technical competence is empty without an understanding of the basis, intent and nature of scientific research ... All else is subordinate to this.

This paradigm of technical rationality in which knowledge of the research process is seen as more important than experiential nursing knowledge is therefore extremely seductive, particularly to beginning nurses, since it implies that we do not need knowledge or experience of a particular practice situation in order to make clinical judgements about it. As the educationalist Stephen Kemmis (1980) put it, it is 'as if research workers could somehow "guarantee" the truth of their findings'. Thus:

> without understanding why one course of action is better than another, we could prove by statistical treatment that it is. The vision is an enticing one: it suggests that we may make wise judgements without understanding what we are doing.
>
> (Stenhouse, 1978)

But of course, Stenhouse was trying to make the point that the 'wise judgements' are not as wise as they first appear, and that our own professional clinical judgement, based on experiential and personal knowledge, should take precedence. But in order to achieve that end, we need somehow to shift the criteria for accepting research findings for our practice from a critique of the methodology of the study to a critique of the findings themselves. As Stenhouse (1985b) continued:

> What I am trying to do is to encourage the feeling that all the statistics can be thrown out if they don't accord with the reality as you know it, and when you look at statistical results, somehow the thing to do is to end up not talking about standard deviations but talking about experience.

This is not to say that Stenhouse was opposed to quantitative research and in favour of a more qualitative approach, but rather that he was against the dominance of the academic research-based paradigm over practice. 'The issue is not qualitative versus quantitative, but samples versus cases, and results versus judgements' (Stenhouse, 1979b). Thus, when faced with a conflict between experiential and scientific knowledge, our professional judgement should take precedence, since it is founded on experience of real clinical situations rather than on statistics gathered from research projects. As Stenhouse (1981) maintained:

> the professional researcher seems to me more vulnerable because of his distance from practice and his lack of responsibility for practice than is the [practitioner] by virtue of his involvement in practice.

Thus, 'researchers must justify themselves to practitioners, not practitioners to researchers', and if research findings do not readily translate into improved practice it is the responsibility of the researcher rather than the practitioner to explain why.[1]

There are two obstacles to Stenhouse's vision of professional judgement overriding research findings. The first problem is that the nursing profession, dominated as it is by academics and researchers, is not prepared to accept the judgement of a practitioner over the findings from scientific research studies. Research is seen as the ultimate arbiter in issues of safe and effective practice, and if we are to convince academics that professional judgement is a sound basis for practice, then we must do so on their terms, that is, through research. Thus:

> If after comparing the measurement results with your own experience you find yourself uncertain of judgement, then basically there's no alternative to doing your own research [in your own practice setting].
>
> (Stenhouse, 1985b)

We can now see why Stenhouse felt strongly that using research means doing research, but this raises a second problem for the practitioner–researcher, since most nurses do not have the time to conduct research, or even to sit down and reflect on their practice. In the quest for efficiency and value for money, issues of quality are often neglected in favour of issues of quantity. Nurses are expected to use their own time to keep up to date with the latest research findings, and to apply those findings unquestioningly to their own practice.

This is clearly an unacceptable situation, but there are two points which need to be made. The first is that, however much or little time she has, one of the duties of the nurse is to strive to improve her practice. It is clear that the scope of nursing is so broad as to preclude the possibility of perfect practice, and therefore there is always room for improvement. And if we accept that professional judgement should play a role in nursing practice, then improvement means not only keeping up to date with the scientific literature, but also constantly updating our experiential knowledge-base. Research which generates experiential knowledge is therefore essential to good practice.

The second point is that this research need not be seen as a substitute for practice, but rather as a component of practice. Stenhouse (1985c) differentiated between a research act and a substantive act:

> A research act is an action to further an enquiry. If you ask someone to explain why he did it, he will answer: to find something out. A substantive act is justified by some change in the world or other people which is judged to be desirable.

The aim of scientific research is to uncover new knowledge and theory and is therefore a 'research act', whereas in practitioner research, 'the research act is necessarily a substantive act; the act of finding out has to be undertaken with an obligation to benefit others than the research community' (Stenhouse, 1985c).

Practitioner research is part of practice, and contributes not only to the generation of personal and experiential knowledge, but towards better nursing care. Practitioner research does not detract from practice, but adds to it. When the nurse researches the way in which she gives information to her patients awaiting surgery, she is not only increasing her store of personal and experiential knowledge, but is experimenting with, and improving, her practice. Furthermore, her research is part of her practice: she is not researching *and then* practising, but is carrying out a single substantive act, a new way of nursing

Part Two of this book is an exposition of this new way. It begins by

outlining the requirements of a practitioner-centred research paradigm and exploring how such a paradigm would differ from the
existing scientific approach to research. It then considers several of
the most fundamental and controversial differences between the two
paradigms, including the issues of generalizability and subjectivity.

This is followed by an exploration of the kinds of questions that
can be addressed by practitioner-centred research, and three particular research needs of the nurse–practitioner are identified, namely
the need for replicative, reflective and reflexive research. The final
three chapters of Part Two expound on practitioner-centred methodologies for meeting those needs.

Notes

1. This is the exact opposite of the attitude dominant in nursing, where the
   failure of research to be translated into practice is usually blamed on the
   practitioner.

3

A new paradigm for the practitioner–researcher

Towards a new paradigm

You might recall from the Introduction to Part One that a paradigm was described as an organizing framework which determines not only the values and philosophy of a discipline, but also the questions that can legitimately be asked within that discipline and the research methods and methodologies that can most effectively answer them. In laying the foundations for a new research paradigm, each of these issues will be explored in turn, starting with the question of the fundamental values which underpin the new paradigm.

Science and history

As we saw in Part One, Stenhouse compared the practitioner to a gardener who is concerned with the individual care of each of her unique plants, and the scientific researcher to a farmer who wants to find the most generally effective treatment for a whole field of crops. It is perhaps no coincidence, then, that social scientists sometimes refer to data collection as 'field work', which conjures up an image of the researcher measuring the effectiveness of, say, a new fertilizer by counting individual ears of corn in a field.

This image can be contrasted with that of the gardener, who lovingly tends her plants, concerned for their individual well-being, and perhaps even talks to them. The practitioner, like the gardener, is concerned with individuals, with relationship building, and with personal and experiential knowledge, in contrast to the scientific researcher's concern with statistical generalizations and scientific knowledge. The gardener cannot trust scientific knowledge because it tells her nothing about the well-being of an individual plant, but only about the gross yield of the whole field.

What the practitioner requires, then, is an approach which allows her not only to carry out research into her own practice in order to generate and verify her experiential and personal knowledge, but also to test out scientific knowledge in her own clinical setting by experimenting at the level of individual patients; in short, a 'science of the singular' (Hamilton, 1980). The traditional scientific research paradigm is clearly inadequate for the task, since it is concerned with the generation of objective generalizable data rather than specific data about specific individuals in specific situations and 'what it yields are indications of trends, that is, actuarial predictions for populations' (Stenhouse, 1981).

As Stenhouse noted, when social scientists and researchers discuss practice, they do so using the language of theory and research, and are primarily concerned not with whether knowledge is applicable or relevant to practice, but with whether it was generated in a scientifically acceptable way and whether it is generalizable. Practitioners, on the other hand, require knowledge that will be effective in individual practice settings, knowledge that is useful to *their* practice rather than generalizable to the practice of others. What is needed, then, is a research paradigm which generates knowledge and theory for practice to complement the existing technical rationality paradigm which provides us with generalizable theory.

Van Manen (1990), writing about teaching rather than nursing, made a similar point:

> Pedagogic situations are always unique. And so, what we need more of is theory not consisting of generalizations, which we then have difficulty applying to concrete and ever-changing circumstances, but *theory of the unique*; that is, theory eminently suitable to deal with this particular pedagogic situation, this school, that child, or this class of youngsters.

In response to the requirements of the practitioner for a theory of the unique, Stenhouse offered what he called the paradigm of history, which is based on personal judgement rather than on the construction of generalizable laws, and is therefore more concerned with practice than with the generation of theory. History, he claimed, is 'the archetypal utilitarian research', such that:

> while the hard sciences produce our hardware, history produces our software: it is the expression of a systematic critical enquiry into the fruits of our experience.
>
> (Stenhouse, 1981)

When he spoke of the paradigm of history, Stenhouse was not referring to historical research, that is, research into the past, but to research that is based on experience rather than on the manipulation and control of variables. Whereas the aim of scientific research is to produce generalizable knowledge, theories and laws, the aim of history is to strengthen professional judgement, that is, to help us to deal with Schön's 'swampy lowland' of practice and the unpredictability of individual cases.

Some researchers might object at this point that there is little difference between what Stenhouse referred to as history and the social science methodology of ethnography, the study of particular social groups, usually by participant observation. However, whereas ethnography is concerned with trying to understand other cultures from an emic perspective, that is, from the 'native's point of view' (Harris, 1968), history is concerned with trying to understand our *own* culture. As Stenhouse put it:

> there is a sense in which history is the work of insiders, ethnography of outsiders. In its origins history has been how the ruling classes write about their own society, ethnography has been how they write about the societies of others.
>
> (Stenhouse, 1984a)

Some social scientists have pointed out that, in recent years, ethnography has 'come home' (Burgess, 1984) and that ethnographers are now just as likely to engage in field research where the focus is their own society as they are to study other cultures. However, they might well be studying their own culture, but they are nevertheless doing so from the perspective of an outsider or an interested observer. They might well be studying their own society, but they are not studying themselves or their impact on that society.

In fact, as we shall see later, ethnographers actively attempt to eliminate the impact that they as researchers might have on the group or society they are studying. And even when that society is familiar to them:

> the participant observer is required to treat it as "anthropologically strange" in an effort to make explicit the assumptions he or she takes for granted as a culture member.
>
> (Hammersley and Atkinson, 1983)

Furthermore, ethnographic approaches, 'while claiming to "tell it like it is" leave the telling to the researcher and do little to challenge the unequal power relationships between researcher and researched'

(Hart, 1996). The essential difference between the soft, interpretive ethnographic end of the traditional scientific research spectrum and the paradigm of history, then, is that traditional science studies others whereas history studies ourselves and, more importantly, our impact on the practice situation. So, for example, when a particular care intervention is assessed from the paradigm of technical rationality, it is usually done so 'objectively' in relation to its outcomes: the social scientist measures or assesses whether the patients received better care from either an external, objective etic perspective, from the viewpoint of an impersonal observer; or from an internal, subjective emic perspective, from the viewpoint of the patients themselves. In either case, however, the influence of the individual practitioner is not sought; on the contrary, the influence of the individual is seen as an extraneous variable, and every effort is made to minimize her impact on the findings.

However, when the paradigm of history is employed to assess a nursing care intervention, it does so from the perspective of a specific nurse or nursing team. The aim is not to produce generalizations by objectively evaluating the care intervention 'scientifically', isolating it from its context and from individual care-givers, but to evaluate how a particular nurse or nursing team utilizes that intervention in a particular setting. The primary aim of the research is not to provide general and generalizable findings about the care intervention, but to evaluate a specific instance in which it was applied. The focus is therefore on the practitioners rather than on the intervention, on how that intervention was given in this particular case and, more importantly, on how it could have been given more effectively.

Generalizable scientific research has its place, and is able to provide us with the 'big picture', with statistical data about what is likely to happen in general, or how the average person would respond in a particular situation. But knowledge and theory about specifics requires the more intimate approach of the paradigm of history. And if history is the work of insiders, and the focus is on what happens in specific situations rather than in general, then clinical research into individualized nursing practice can best (and perhaps only) be carried out by nurses themselves.

The 'new paradigm' or cooperative inquiry school of research went some way towards realizing this aim by calling for research in which researchers and researched work together in an equal partnership (Reason and Rowan, 1981; Reason, 1988), but the challenge of finding ways to carry out research into ourselves and our own impact on the practice setting has been taken up most enthusiastically by the discipline of education, where it is usually referred to as practitioner-based enquiry.

However, all of these terms are potentially misleading: 'history' is easily confused with historical research, 'new paradigm' research is no longer new, and 'practitioner-based enquiry' does not capture the full flavour of the practitioner researching her own practice. For example, Fuller and Petch (1995), writing about practitioner-based enquiry in social work, took it to mean:

> simply research undertaken by practitioners; we intend no implication in principle that particular research approaches, strategies or methods will be used by practitioner–researchers, or that a particular style of research characterizes their efforts.

According to this definition, practitioner-based enquiry falls far short of an alternative research paradigm, and is distinguished from traditional scientific research only by the person conducting it.

In contrast, I prefer the term 'practitioner-centred research' (PCR) to refer to what is, in effect, an alternative paradigm to technical rationality. It is practitioner-*centred* rather than practitioner-based because it is research undertaken by the practitioner *into herself and her own practice*; and it is research rather than enquiry to emphasize the point that it should be seen as a serious alternative to the traditional scientific research paradigm. Stenhouse offered a very useful 'minimal definition' of research which perfectly describes PCR. Thus, for our purposes: *practitioner-centred research is systematic self-critical enquiry made public.* It is a systematic process of generating knowledge, theory and practice, focused on itself and disseminated to a wider audience.

It can be seen from the above discussion, then, that PCR is concerned with the practitioner examining herself, her attitudes and her practice, and it therefore introduces the concept of the practitioner–researcher. And because the researcher is also the practitioner whose work is being researched, it is essentially a reflexive approach in which the research has a direct impact on the practice, which in turn modifies the research, and so on. This introspective, subjective perspective contrasts strikingly with the detached, objective approach of the scientific paradigm of technical-rationality, and practitioner-centred research is therefore fundamentally different from traditional scientific research. It is not merely that PCR involves practitioners in the research process, but, rather, that it is a distinct type of research with a different philosophy, different aims, different methods and different outcomes from scientific research.

PCR does not reject social science research and the technical rationality paradigm, but offers an alternative and complementary approach, more suited to generating knowledge and theory for individualized practice. It does not argue that scientific research is of no use to nursing, but that there is more to nursing practice than the application of scientific research findings.

In addition, it does not dismiss macro theory generation and scientific knowledge as inappropriate goals for nursing research, but claims that micro theory, personal knowledge and clinical change are at least as important, and that meaningful clinical change can only be assured by involving practitioners in researching their own practice, and by designing research studies which have built-in mechanisms for directly improving practice.

Traditional scientific research is still necessary, and there are, in fact, a number of distinct areas of research where the technical rationality paradigm is more appropriate than PCR: first, in the construction of generalizable nursing theory; secondly, in answering actuarial questions about the statistical effectiveness of various nursing interventions; and thirdly, in the study of generalized group behaviour. However, if we wish to generate knowledge and theory which can be applied to specific patients in specific clinical settings, then those patients and those settings must be incorporated into the research design, that is, it must take a micro, practitioner-centred approach. Now turn to the Reflective Break on page 77.

The fundamental difference between these two approaches, generalizable theoretical research on the one hand and individualized practitioner-centred research on the other, can be seen in the way that each approach deals with the relationship between research and practice (Figure 3.1).

The most noticeable distinction between the two is that in PCR the entire level of theory-building is absent. Whereas the knowledge generated from scientific research is employed to build inductively generalizable theory, the knowledge generated from PCR is applied directly to practice. Furthermore, practice is not seen as the end-product of PCR, but as the spring-board for further research. Thus, practitioner-centred research is generated *from* practice and immediately applied back *to* practice in a reflexive cycle.

This fundamental difference between scientific research based on the technical rationality paradigm and PCR highlights some important contrasts in their values and philosophies, particularly their attitudes towards generalizability and objectivity. These are both complex issues, and each merits a detailed discussion.

REFLECTIVE BREAK

PROFESSIONAL JUDGEMENT AND PRACTITIONER-CENTRED RESEARCH

Think back to the situation you described in the Reflective Break on page 62. How could practitioner-centred research have helped you to test out and verify your professional judgement?

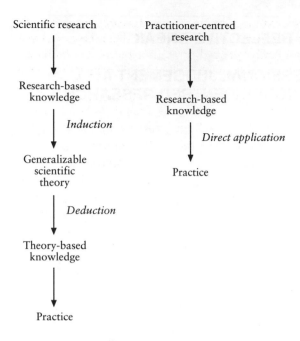

Figure 3.1   *The relationship between research and practice in scientific research and practitioner-centred research.*

Generalizability

Practitioner-centred research is primarily concerned with generating personal knowledge about the practitioner herself and her impact on individual patients, and so the issue of generalizing the findings to other practitioners, patients or groups of patients might not appear to be relevant. But PCR is also concerned with the generation of experiential knowledge, that is, of clusters of paradigm cases around a specific clinical issue, and it is important that these cases stand in some sort of relationship to one another and are not merely a collection of unrelated and isolated examples. It is therefore essential that the knowledge obtained from PCR is able to be generalized to other cases.

However, we have already seen that the kind of statistical generalization usually employed in the social sciences and medicine cannot tell us anything about the needs of individual patients. What is required, then, is a different kind of generalizability, one more suited to the small-scale personal nature of PCR.

This issue has been explored by qualitative researchers, for whom generalizability depends largely on the contextual similarity between two settings, and is usually referred to as transferability (Guba and Lincoln, 1989) or fittingness (Sandelowski, 1986; Koch, 1994). Thus:

> a study meets the criterion of fittingness when its findings can "fit" into contexts outside the study situation and when its audience views its findings as meaningful and applicable in terms of their own experiences.
>
> (Sandelowski, 1986)

By employing the notion of fittingness, the personal knowledge obtained from working with one particular patient can be employed with other patients, provided that the context is sufficiently similar. In this way, personal knowledge can cluster and accumulate into experiential knowledge, but the implication of fittingness is that experiential knowledge, like personal knowledge, is context-specific.

For example, the personal knowledge gained by the practitioner–researcher from researching her practice with each of six individual patients who have attempted suicide can be accumulated into experiential knowledge about the way she works with these kinds of patients in general. However, all six cases must be similar in context, and the experiential knowledge which she has generated can only be transferred to her work with other patients in the same setting.

In reporting practitioner-centred research, then, 'the original context must be described adequately so that a judgement of transferability can be made by the readers' (Koch, 1994). The concept of fittingness also opens up the possibility that personal knowledge is transferable between practitioners, and that the personal knowledge of one practitioner–researcher can be employed by another in a similar situation. Stake (1980) referred to this as naturalistic generalization, 'arrived at by recognizing the similarities of objects and issues in and out of context and by sensing the natural covariations of happenings'.

There is, however, yet another form of generalizability that is relevant to PCR. Yin (1994) distinguished between statistical generalization, that is, generalizing from a sample to a population which the sample is said to represent; and analytic generalization, that is, generalizing from a single case to a theoretical proposition, where 'the investigator's goal is to expand and generalize theories and not to enumerate frequencies' (Yin, 1994). The purpose of analytic generalization, then, is to employ single cases to construct and test theories.

Analytic generalization is the logical mechanism employed in the classic form of the scientific experiment. For example, the theory that water boils at 100 degrees Celsius can be tested by a single experiment of heating up a test-tube of water and noting its boiling point. The scientist does not boil up 50 test-tubes and compute the average, since if the experiment is performed properly, she will obtain the same result every time. If the experiment *is* repeated, it takes the form of a replication which strengthens her confidence in the theory. The experimenter is not *repeating* the experiment with a different subject in order to extend the population to which a statistical generalization can be made, but *replicating* the experiment in order to add weight to the theory being tested.

This concept of analytic generalization allows the practitioner–researcher not only to apply the findings from one case to other cases in similar contexts, but to generalize to other contexts and patient groups. For example, she might wish to explore the effectiveness of a particular form of counselling. The first step would be to construct a theory based on her existing personal and experiential knowledge, for example, that her counselling intervention will be effective with middle-aged men. She then attempts to test her theory by assessing the effects of the counselling intervention on one particular middle-aged male patient. If he responds to the treatment, the practitioner–researcher has some grounds for accepting the theory and for applying it to other similar patients.

By successfully replicating the study with other middle-aged male patients, the theory is strengthened, but like the water-boiling experiment, the aim is not to pool the findings and find an average but to add weight to the theory. If, on the other hand, the intervention is unsuccessful with other patients, then the theory is too broad, and needs to be reformulated. As Shontz (1965) noted:

> The investigator will be in a position either to modify his thinking or to state more clearly the conditions under which the hypothesis does and does not provide a useful model of psychological events.

By examining the differences between the patients for whom the intervention is successful and those for whom it is not, the practitioner–researcher might find, for example, that hair colour appears to be a factor, and so her new theory might be that her counselling intervention will be effective with middle-aged blond men.

The theory can then be expanded by repeating the study in a variety of different settings and with a variety of different patients, for example, with female patients or with younger people. In this way, a very precise picture can be built up of those specific groups of patients for whom the treatment is effective. As Barlow and Hersen (1984) pointed out:

> the more we learn about the effects of a treatment on different individuals, in different settings, and so on, the easier it will be to determine if that treatment will be effective with the next individual walking into the office.

By carrying out a series of carefully selected studies of individual patients, the practitioner–researcher can therefore formulate theories that are generalizable to other patients. But they are not theories based on statistics, and are not subject to the same problems of generalizability as traditional scientific theories.[1]

The golden rule of analytic generalization is never to generalize outside of the particular variables present in the patient we are working with. Just as we cannot generalize to the boiling point of milk from the boiling point of water, so we cannot generalize from the effectiveness of an intervention with middle-aged men to its effectiveness with young women. The art of formulating theories for PCR is therefore in knowing which variables are likely to have an influence on the treatment intervention. If we believe that hair colour has no effect on treatment, then there is no point in wasting our time controlling for it. As Barlow and Hersen (who used the term 'logical generalization' for what Yin referred to as analytic generalization) pointed out:

> The process of logical generalization depends on similarities between the patient in the homogeneous group and the individual in question in the clinician's office. Which features of a case are important for extending logical generalization and which features can be ignored (eg, hair colour) will depend on the judgement of the clinician and the state of knowledge at the time.
>
> (Barlow and Hersen, 1984)

The professional judgement of the nurse, that is, a combination of her scientific, personal and experiential knowledge, is therefore essential in the formulation of the theory to be tested. It is possible to generalize from the findings of small-scale, and even from single-case, practitioner-centred research, but to do so requires a store of experiential knowledge.

The psychologist and educationalist Carl Rogers made a similar claim that the researcher must immerse herself in the practice situation she is attempting to explore, and:

> Out of this complete subjective immersion comes a creative forming, a sense of direction, a vague formulation of relationships hitherto unrecognised. Whittled down, sharpened, formulated in clearer terms, this creative forming becomes a hypothesis – a statement of a tentative, personal, subjective faith.
>
> (Rogers, 1956)

Unlike traditional scientific research, therefore, the clinically inexperienced, disinterested academic researcher cannot carry out effective PCR, since she cannot attain 'complete subjective immersion' in the practice situation and does not possess the required professional judgement necessary for theory generation.

To summarize, PCR rejects the traditional scientific notion of statistical generalizability as inappropriate for research into specific clinical situations, but this should not be taken to mean that the findings from PCR are not generalizable. First, we can borrow the concept of naturalistic generalization in order to extend the findings from a clinical encounter between a practitioner and a patient to encounters between that practitioner and other patients, and even to other practitioners, provided that the clinical context is sufficiently similar. And secondly, we can employ analytic generalizations to build theories based on professional judgements from a series of carefully chosen individual cases.

Subjectivity and prejudice

The second major difference between scientific research and PCR to be discussed is the issue of subjectivity. It is now widely recognized that science cannot escape subjectivity. Indeed, recent post-modern critiques argue not only that the methods of science are inescapably subjective, but that science itself is merely one of an infinite number of 'world views'. From this perspective, science cannot claim to be the only, or even the best, method of generating knowledge, and the knowledge that it produces cannot be claimed to be either more or less 'objective' than the knowledge generated by any other method.

Even in the 'hard' physical sciences, which have traditionally promoted the scientist as a detached figure in a white coat, standing outside of the situation which she is seeking to measure, there is a growing recognition of the degree to which the researcher must inevitably become involved with what she is studying. As the eminent physicist Werner Heisenberg (1963) pointed out: 'natural science does not simply describe and explain nature; it is part of the interplay between nature and ourselves'. He continued: 'the conventional division of the world into subject and object, into inner and outer world, into body and soul, is no longer applicable'. Thus:

> In atomic physics, then, the scientist cannot play the role of the detached observer, but becomes involved in the world he observes to the extent that he influences the properties of the observed subjects.
>
> (Capra, 1976)

And if the physicist cannot detach herself from what she is observing, how much more difficult for the social scientist, who is investigating the behaviour of thinking, reacting people who 'are fully capable of adjusting their behaviour and the meaning they give to events if a social scientist starts to investigate their lives' (Shipman, 1972).

However rigorously the research study is designed and conducted, the introduction of subjective bias is inevitable, either at the data collection stage or at the stage of interpreting the data as knowledge, and as Sandelowski (1986) pointed out, 'objectivity is itself a socially constructed phenomenon that produces the illusion of objectivity'. All knowledge is therefore subjectively constructed by human beings, and

> research is not a process of thought going out to embrace its object as if its object lay there inert, waiting to be discovered
>
> (Kemmis, 1980).

Rather, 'each researcher sees research findings through her own personal theoretical "lens"' (Schutz, 1994).

However, while many social scientists and nurse researchers now accept as inevitable the subjective nature of scientific enquiry, most see it as something undesirable, and attempt to minimize its effect on their research findings. Phenomenologists talk of suspending or 'bracketing' their beliefs and preconceptions during the research process, whereas Schutz (1994) argued that 'it is the skill and experience of the researcher as an individual, in interpretation and understanding, that will overcome bias and prejudice'. The prevailing view is that the subjectivity inherent in the research process must somehow be overcome, and that it can only be overcome if it is first of all acknowledged.

Practitioner-centred research, however, is not merely arguing that subjectivity is inevitable, but that it is desirable, and even *essential* if research is to improve practice. Stenhouse (1981) believed that to ask whether the researcher was subjectively biased was to ask the wrong question. The issue is not one of values, but of *interest*, in both its dictionary definitions. The practitioner–researcher should therefore have a personal interest in what she is researching, first by being 'concerned or affected in respect of advantage or detriment'; and secondly by possessing 'feeling of concern for or curiosity about a person or thing'.

For Stenhouse, then, the practitioner–researcher will have an interest in, or concern about, what she is researching, but will also choose to carry out research that is in her best interest. Thus:

> we build a bridge because it is advantageous to us to do so and that advantage breeds a curiosity about bridges. Moreover, the building of a good bridge is to our advantage not only in the primary sense that it lets us cross the river, but also in the secondary sense that successful achievement rewards us in terms of reputation, material payment and future opportunities.
>
> (Stenhouse, 1981)

We do not design and build bridges simply for fun or because we have nothing better to do, we build them primarily because we have a practical interest in crossing a river, but also in furthering our own professional ends. To pretend that we are completely objective and disinterested as to where the bridge is to be sited and how well it is constructed is not only naive but dangerous. We always have a point of view, and we are usually motivated by the thought of making the world a better place, both for us and for others. The question, then, is not whether we should take sides, but whose side we should take.

Gadamer (1976) referred to this interest as 'prejudice', which should be seen in a positive way: 'prejudice is our situatedness in history and time – is the precondition of truth, not an obstacle to it' (Thompson, 1990). We take sides according to our prejudice, according to our values, and 'these values, rather than getting in the way of research, make research meaningful' (Koch, 1994). And the most important values of the practitioner–researcher are her values about how practice might be done better. The nurse who is researching her own practice does not merely want to bring about change; she wants to bring about improvements, and that entails making a subjective value-judgement, what Reason (1988) termed 'critical subjectivity'. As Schön (1983) pointed out, the practitioner–researcher 'has an interest in transforming the situation from what it is to something he likes better'.

To summarize, there is a growing awareness not only in the social sciences, but also in the hard physical sciences, of the inevitable subjectivity implicit in the research process and hence in the product of research. Scientific knowledge is, to a greater or lesser extent, subjective and constructed by the researcher. However, whilst recognizing this subjectivity, the aim of technical rationality is to transcend or overcome it: it is seen as an inevitable barrier to generalizable knowledge, and the idiosyncratic perspective or influence of the individual researcher must, as far as possible, be bracketed off or screened out. In contrast to this view, PCR welcomes the 'prejudice' of the practitioner–researcher as an essential component of the research process if the product of that research is to be improvement rather than mere change. Now look at the Reflective Break on page 86.

Beyond method

If we accept the argument expressed earlier by Kemmis that knowledge is constructed rather than uncovered, then the role of the practitioner–researcher is not one of discovery but of creation, and research takes on many of the features of an art rather than a science. As Sandelowski (1986) observed:

> The artistic approach to qualitative enquiry emphasizes the irreplicability of the research process and product. The artistic integrity, rather than the scientific objectivity, of the research is achieved when the researcher communicates the richness and diversity of human experience in an engaging and even poetic manner.

The research act is unique and unrepeatable, and as such is more akin to artistic creation than to a formal structured process. Stenhouse (1984b) applied this view to practitioner-centred research, stating that 'the artist is the researcher whose enquiry expresses itself in the performance of his art rather than (or as well as) in a research report'. In other words, the aim of practitioner-centred research is to improve performance, indeed, research that is conducted by academics away from the practice setting and which is not immediately translated into improved practice is like 'so many theatres without players, galleries without pictures, music without musicians' (Stenhouse, 1984b).

And like the artist or the musician, the researcher should be *guided* by rules and methods rather than bound by them. The novice artist or musician, like the novice researcher, needs rules to guide her art, but the skill of a great artist is in knowing when the rules should be broken. Similarly in effective research, 'there is not a single rule, however plausible, and however firmly grounded in epistemology, that is not violated at some time or other' (Feyerabend, 1970).

But more than this, creativity *demands* that we bend or break the rules. Giorgi (1971) claimed that 'method frequently interferes with

---

REFLECTIVE BREAK

EXPLORING YOUR PREJUDICE

Think back again to the situation you described in the Reflective Breaks on pages 62 and 77. What preconceived ideas did you bring to that situation?

Now think about your interest in the situation. What was your practical interest in it?

What was your professional interest?

---

meaning', whilst the philosopher Roland Barthes observed that 'some people speak of method greedily, demandingly; what they want in work is method; to them it never seems rigorous enough, formal enough. Method becomes a Law'. But, he continued:

> The invariable fact is that a work which constantly proclaims its will-to-method is ultimately sterile: everything has to be put into the method, nothing remains for the writing; the researcher insists that his text will be methodological, but this text never comes: no surer way to kill a piece of research and send it to join the great scrap heap of abandoned projects than Method.
>
> (Barthes, 1986)

For Barthes, the creativity demanded of writing the research is stifled by method. Thus, 'at a certain moment, therefore, it is necessary to turn against method, or at least to treat it without any founding privilege as one of the voices of plurality'.

A similar point was made by Feyerabend (1970), that:

> One of the most striking features of recent discussions in the history and philosophy of science is the realisation that developments ... occurred either because some thinkers decided not to be bound by certain "obvious" methodological rules or because they unwittingly broke them.

The scientific, technical rationality paradigm does not acknowledge this deliberate flaunting of the rules of research, since for most scientists, research *is* method. However, even Einstein recognized the constraining force of the traditional scientific method when he wrote:

> The external conditions which are set for [the scientist] by the facts of experience do not permit him to let himself be too much restricted in the construction of his conceptual world by the adherence to an epistemological system. He therefore must appear to the systematic epistemologist as a type of unscrupulous opportunist.
>
> (cited in Schlipp, 1948)

The rigorous application of established and accepted method brings with it the promise of validity essential for findings that are to be generalized beyond the sample from which they were taken, but at the same time it severely limits the scope of what that research can achieve. PCR is not concerned with statistical generalizability, and is therefore not constrained by the limitations imposed by the rigorous and unbending application of established methods.

That is not to say, however, that PCR eschews all the rules, but that it constructs its own, albeit flexible, methodologies; methodologies which are designed to meet the practice-centred aims of the practitioner–researcher. PCR is not rule-bound, but, you might recall, is '*systematic* self-critical enquiry made public'.

Asking practitioner-centred research questions

Having explored some of the underlying issues concerning the values and philosophy of PCR, I will now turn my attention to the kinds of questions that can legitimately be asked. Any research paradigm will be oriented towards answering particular kinds of questions. Technical rationality is best suited to questions which seek to uncover knowledge and build theory about the world in general, and about how certain categories of people tend to behave in particular situations. PCR, on the other hand, seeks to find answers to questions about the researcher's own practice, questions about the clinical environment in which she works, and even questions about her own personal qualities, beliefs and philosophy of care. Thus, whereas the paradigm of technical rationality adopts an outward-looking perspective and a separation between the researcher and her research subjects, PCR is inward-looking and introspective and combines researcher and subject in the person of the practitioner–researcher.

In order to impose a structure on this exploration of the questions addressed by PCR, I have attempted to construct a typology with three dimensions, namely, the *form* of the question to be asked, its *focus*, and its *subject*.

The form of the question

The form that the question takes determines whether it seeks to describe, explain or bring about change, and follows much the same format in PCR as it does in traditional scientific research.

Descriptive questions attempt to understand or describe a situation, usually by establishing relationships between variables. They are often 'what' questions, for example: *what is the relationship between pre-operative information giving and post-operative recovery?* These questions often require the generation of statistical data.

Exploratory questions explain or explore an issue, usually a previously established relationship. They tend to be 'why' questions, for example: *why is there a relationship between pre-operative informa-*

tion giving and post-operative recovery? These questions usually require the generation of qualitative data.

Developmental questions attempt to change or improve a situation, usually in well-researched areas. They are nearly always 'how' questions, for example: *how can we modify the information we give to patients in order to improve post-operative recovery?* These questions usually require an approach which includes an action component.

It can be seen that these three forms of question follow a natural sequence: we cannot ask a developmental question until we have answered an exploratory question, and we cannot ask an exploratory question until we have answered a descriptive question. Until we have established that a relationship exists between pre-operative information-giving and post-operative recovery, we cannot explore that relationship. And until we have explored that relationship and understand it intimately, we cannot improve it.

The focus of the question

The focus of the question determines who or what it is directed at, and this is where the two paradigms go their separate ways. Whereas technical rationality usually focuses on the outside world and maintains a distinction between the researcher and the research, the focus of PCR is on the practitioner–researcher herself, on her clinical work and on the way that she manages herself and her time.

Introspective questions focus on the self as a therapeutic agent. They might be concerned with exploring the practitioner–researcher's personal philosophy of care, beliefs and attitudes, or with exploring her personal qualities, skills, knowledge and expertise.

Practice-based questions focus on the practitioner–researcher's clinical work; on her relationships with patients, on the effectiveness of clinical interventions, or on models and strategies of practice.

Organizational questions focus on care management issues, for example, the organization of care, time and resources.

The subject of the question

The subject of the question relates to the setting of the research and its relationship to the outside world. Technical rationality research usually aims to be generalizable, and so its subject is broader than the sample of people or things being studied. It might, for example, be nurses in general, hospitals in general or, indeed, the entire population of a country. And because the population to which the findings are to be generalized is often very large and heterogeneous, the sample itself is usually fairly extensive.

PCR, on the other hand, is not concerned with statistical generalizability, and confines itself to the practitioner–researcher herself and to her working environment. It is therefore small-scale, local, and relates either to the practitioner herself or to her immediate environment.

Personal questions relate to the practitioner–researcher's own practice.

Environmental questions relate to her working environment.

These three aspects of the research question – its form, its focus and its subject – can be combined in a three-dimensional table to produce 18 different kinds of questions that PCR can address (Figure 3.2).

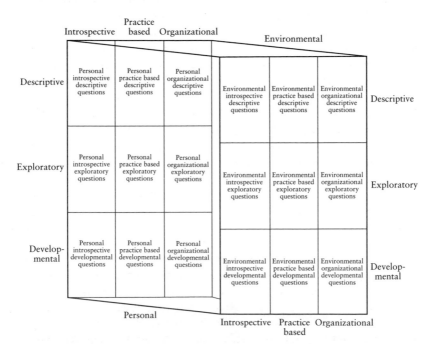

Figure 3.2   *Practitioner-centred research questions.*

We shall now look at some actual examples of practitioner-centred research questions. First, we shall formulate a personal, practice-based, descriptive question, for example: *what would be the effect of introducing a new treatment for leg ulcers into my nursing care?* We can see that this question is personal because it relates to the practitioner–researcher herself; it is practice-based because it focuses on her clinical work, and in particular, on the effectiveness of a particular clinical intervention; and it is a descriptive question which seeks to establish a relationship between a new treatment and a measure of clinical outcome. It is the sort of question that a practitioner–researcher might ask in order to evaluate the effectiveness of the findings of a scientific research study for her own practice.

Secondly, we shall formulate an environmental, organizational, exploratory question, for example: *why does my ward not allow open visiting?* This question is environmental because it relates not directly to the practitioner–researcher but to her working environment; it is organizational because it is concerned with the organization of time and resources; and it is exploratory because it seeks to explore an established practice in greater detail. It is the kind of question that a practitioner–researcher might ask in order to explore and challenge the way that care is organized and delivered on her ward.

Now let us construct a personal, introspective, exploratory question, for example: *why do I become angry with patients who attempt to commit suicide?* We can see that this question is personal because it relates to the practitioner–researcher's own practice; it is introspective by focusing on herself and her feelings and attitudes; and it is an exploratory question which seeks to explore the well-established issue of her anger towards certain of her patients. It is the kind of question that a practitioner–researcher might ask as part of her reflection-on-action, possibly during clinical supervision.

Furthermore, it leads on naturally to a personal, introspective, developmental question such as: *how can I become less angry with these patients?* This question can only be asked once the exploratory question has been answered, and seeks to improve the way that the practitioner–researcher relates to her patients. It is a question that she might ask as part of her reflection-in-action.

Finally, let us formulate a personal, organizational, developmental question, such as: *how can I re-organize my time to provide better individualized care to my patients?* This question is personal because it relates to the practitioner–researcher's own practice; it is organizational because it focuses on how she organizes her time; and it is a developmental question which seeks to change the way that she does things. It is the kind of question that a practitioner–researcher might ask as the first step in improving her practice through PCR.

We shall return to each of these questions later in the chapter. Now look at the Reflective Break on page 93.

Methodologies for practitioner-centred research

We have seen that the purpose of PCR is to generate personal and experiential knowledge for and about the practitioner–researcher herself, and it is possible to identify a number of different research needs arising directly from her clinical practice.

First, the practitioner–researcher requires a way of verifying the findings and recommendations of scientific research for her own practice with her own patients. In other words, she needs to be able to resolve the conflict between her professional judgement and the findings of scientific research by testing out those findings in her own practice setting with her own patients.

Secondly, the practitioner–researcher needs a way not only of generating a store of personal knowledge about herself and her individual patients, and experiential knowledge about situations similar to the one she now finds herself in, but also of testing out the personal theories constructed from that knowledge.

Thirdly, the practitioner–researcher needs, wherever possible, to be able to integrate her research into her everyday practice, so that practice and research become a single act. We can see, then, that practitioner-centred research can be of three kinds, which I have called replicative, reflective and reflexive research, and which are described below.[2]

Replicative research tests out the findings from generalizable scientific studies in the practitioner–researcher's own clinical area with her own patients, and also attempts to verify the personal theories derived from her personal and experiential knowledge. It is important to note that the aim of replicative research is not to replicate the *methods* of the original study, but to replicate the *findings* in the practitioner–researcher's own clinical setting. Stenhouse referred to this as situational verification, and it is essential if the practitioner wishes her professional judgements to be accepted by the scientific community.

REFLECTIVE BREAK

CONSTRUCTING PRACTITIONER-CENTRED RESEARCH QUESTIONS

Now think of some questions of your own, based on your own practice:

1. A personal organizational descriptive question.

2. A personal organizational exploratory question.

3. An environmental introspective exploratory question.

4. An environmental introspective developmental question.

5. An environmental practice-based developmental question.

Reflective research generates personal and experiential knowledge and theories from the practitioner–researcher's own practice. The aim is not merely to replicate existing findings, but to create new knowledge and theory through a formalized approach to reflection-on-action.

Reflexive research attempts to bring about an integration of practice and research in a single act. The aim here is not the generation of knowledge, which might nevertheless occur as a by-product of the research, but the implementation of clinical change directly through the research process itself.

Each of these three distinct kinds of research requires its own methodology,[3] but unfortunately most traditional technical rationality methodologies were devised to produce generalizable knowledge and theory and are therefore unsuitable for the purposes of PCR. This can be seen most clearly in the case of the more quantitative methodologies such as randomized controlled trials and surveys, which both rely on the accumulation and statistical manipulation of data from representative samples. Even at the qualitative end of the spectrum, approaches such as phenomenology still entail the pooling of data from several respondents to construct generalizable categories and units of meaning.

However, some research methodologies have been developed in partial or total opposition to the ethos of generalizability, and three of these will be adopted for use in PCR, either as they stand or in a modified form. The three that have been chosen are single-case experiments for replicative research, case studies for reflective research and action research for reflexive research. These methodologies do not exist in watertight categories, and there is some overlap between them. For example, although the main use of single-case experiments is to test theories deductively (replicative research), they can also be employed inductively to construct new ones (reflective research). Furthermore, these are not the only methodologies that are suitable for the three kinds of research outlined above, and it is possible that others could be adapted for PCR. Nevertheless, these three methodologies adequately meet the needs of the practitioner–researcher who wishes to explore her own practice.

I will now give a number of simple examples, using the research questions generated earlier, of how these research methodologies can be employed by the practitioner–researcher to generate the kinds of personal and experiential knowledge and theory relevant to her practice.

Single-case experimental research

Single-case experimental research (SCER), which Stenhouse (1984a) has described as the 'systematization of experience', is a particularly effective way for the practitioner–researcher to test the usefulness of a generalizable practice-based theory on her own patients. Even the positivist researcher and statistician Cronbach (1975) claimed that 'when we give proper weight to local conditions, any generalization is a working hypothesis, not a conclusion', implying that generalizable findings from scientific research should form the starting point for local studies rather than an end in themselves.

So, for example, a paper reporting on research into a new treatment for leg ulcers might conclude that it results in significant improvements in 90 per cent of all cases. What the practitioner-researcher is concerned about, however, is whether it will be effective in her clinical area with her patients, or whether they will fall in the 10 per cent who do not improve.

Employing the methodology of single-case experimental research, she might take baseline measures of a particular patient's leg ulcer over a period of a week whilst giving her usual treatment, and then continue to take measures whilst giving the new treatment. If the condition of the ulcer improves under the new treatment compared with the old, then she can surmise that it is effective with this particular patient, and more importantly, she can analytically generalize to a theory about similar patients under similar conditions. She can then strengthen her theory by replicating the experiment with a similar patient under similar conditions, and extend it by replicating with different patients under different conditions. In this way, an elaborate theory can be built up about the kinds of patients and conditions that the new treatment is effective with.

As well as exploring the limits of other people's research, the nurse can also employ this method to test theories based on her own experiential and personal knowledge. However, this simple baseline-treatment (A-B) design has a number of flaws, and is only one of many forms of more elaborate and more effective single-case experimental designs which will be explored in the next chapter.

Case-study research

Benner claimed that the accumulation of experiential knowledge, what she referred to as paradigm cases, is a largely unconscious process which occurs mainly by chance. Case-study research offers the practitioner–researcher a systematic and methodical way not only of generating personal and experiential knowledge, but also of inductively building her own theories.

Case-study research is a formal method of collecting data on a single case from a wide range of perspectives and sources. For example, in order to discover why her ward does not allow open visiting, the practitioner–researcher might conduct interviews, observe practice, consult minutes from meetings and collect statistical data. However, case-study methodology is not merely descriptive, and like the single-case experimental approach, its aim is also to develop a theory or test a hypothesis.

Unlike traditional case-study methodology, where the 'case' and the researcher are clearly distinguished, PCR is introspective and focuses on the nurse researching her own practice. Thus, whereas traditionally the most important and useful case study method is participant or non-participant observation of an external case, in PCR the central method is self-observation or reflection-on-action.

Reflection-on-action, or reflective practice as it is often called, is becoming increasingly popular as more nurses turn to clinical supervision. However, clinical supervision rarely meets the criteria for PCR because it is not usually undertaken in a systematic fashion and is seldom recorded or disseminated to a wider audience. In order for reflection-on-action to be acceptable as PCR, it must therefore be systematically undertaken and recorded and be potentially available for other practitioners to learn from.

The simplest way that this can be achieved is through keeping a reflective diary or through written critical incident analysis. However, as cases and critical incidents accrue, it is necessary to categorize and group them around particular clinical situations according to the process of naturalistic generalization described earlier, and this requires a consideration of not only what happened yesterday, but of what happened last month and last year. In order for reflection-on-action to be a formal and potentially useful method of PCR, it must therefore involve not only the collection of current data, but the analysis and categorization of past data from a variety of perspectives.

For example, in trying to understand why she becomes angry with patients who have attempted suicide, the practitioner–researcher might reflect on her experiences with current patients, recall past experiences, and analyse and categorize this personal knowledge of individual cases into a body of experiential knowledge from which she can then construct personal theories. Formal reflection-on-action can therefore be seen as a powerful method of reflective case-study research, in which the subject is herself and her clinical practice, and which includes diary keeping, clinical supervision, and other reflective techniques in addition to the more traditional forms of case-study data collection such as interviews and document analysis.

Action research

Reflexive research is research which directly influences practice, and action research is one of the few methodologies in which the process of carrying out the research has an immediate impact on the situation being studied. We shall see later that there are a number of conflicting views about the nature of action research, but the model which comes closest to the reflexive approach advocated in this book is that described by McNiff *et al.* (1996). For them, action research is different from other research because:

- it requires action as an integral part of the research process itself;
- it is focused by the researcher's professional values rather than methodological considerations;
- it is necessarily insider research, in the sense of practitioners researching their own professional actions.

(McNiff *et al.*, 1996)

We can see, then, that there are two factors which distinguish action research from the other methodologies described above. First, it is carried out as part of nursing practice rather than being a separate activity. Secondly, it forms with practice a reflexive cycle in which theory is generated from practice, the testing of that theory brings about changes to practice, those changes in turn produce new theory, and so on.

For example, in order to reorganize her time to provide better individualized care to her patients, the practitioner–researcher might decide to change her shift pattern to work more night duties when a particular patient experiences increased distress. She can then evaluate the effect of her intervention by comparing distress levels before and after the change, and modify her shift pattern accordingly. By constantly monitoring and modifying her response, she can fine-tune it to meet the precise needs of her patient. Thus, not only has she generated personal knowledge about the care needs of an individual patient, but she has also implemented a successful nursing intervention.

This form of action research should not be confused with single-case experimental methodology of the simple A-B type discussed earlier. A single-case experiment is concerned with evaluating a new intervention in order to decide whether or not it is appropriate for a particular clinical situation. Action research, on the other hand, is concerned with developing and refining an intervention by constantly modifying it in response to research findings. The former is about evaluating *change*, the latter is about introducing *improvements*.

Although action research is on the fringes of technical rationality, the methods employed are usually fairly traditional and can be either quantitative or qualitative. In the above case, for example, the measurement of stress levels could have involved a quantitative measure such as a structured questionnaire or inventory, or a qualitative semistructured interview.

There is, however, another form of action research which does not employ traditional research methods, and that is Schön's reflection-in-action or on-the-spot experimenting, in which personal theories are formed, tested, modified, re-tested and so on, in direct response to the minute-by-minute demands of practice. Reflection-in-action cannot be planned in advance, but nevertheless qualifies as action research because it not only tests out theory but also modifies and improves practice in an ongoing reflexive cycle.

For example, having reached an understanding of why she becomes angry with her suicidal patients, the practitioner–researcher might now wish to do something to improve the situation. When confronted with her next patient, she might construct a personal theory on the spot which uses the experiential knowledge gained through reflection-on-action, her personal knowledge about this particular patient and about herself and her reaction to such patients, and her scientific knowledge about psychotherapy. This personal theory might be that her angry response is a reaction formation against her real feelings of distress, with the hypothesis that if she shares her distress with her patient, then he might begin to understand first the impact of his actions on others, and secondly that somebody cares about him. This hypothesis can then be tested, and the theory accepted, rejected or modified accordingly.

For the purpose of this book, then, reflection-in-action will be considered as a particularly powerful method of action research in the same way that reflection-on-action was seen as a method of case-study research.

Summary

We saw in the introduction to Part One that a paradigm embodies the beliefs, values and principles of the community of practitioners and academics that espouses it, as well as determining what counts as knowledge and how that knowledge is generated and disseminated. The development of the profession of nursing as an academic discipline has been led mainly by nurse teachers and lecturers, and so it is not surprising that this group has played a major role in determining the paradigm within which nursing operates.

The problem, as we have seen, is that teaching and nursing are two different disciplines, each with its own agenda: the aim of nursing is to provide the best possible care for patients, whereas the aim of teaching is to develop knowledge and skills in students to enable *them* to provide patient care (Jarvis, 1983). Teachers of nursing might *say* that their aim is to improve practice, but that is rather like a teacher of engineering claiming that her aim is to build bridges.

Furthermore, I have argued that teachers and academics tend to value generalizable scientific knowledge, knowledge that has something to say to groups of students about nursing in general and which is easily transmitted from teacher to student. This preference for generalizable knowledge is reflected in the sort of research that teachers and academics normally undertake, and is particularly well suited to the paradigm of technical rationality, which has become the dominant paradigm in nursing.

Practising nurses, however, quickly run up against the limitations of generalizable scientific knowledge, and require personal and experiential knowledge about specific clinical situations with specific patients. The problem is that the personal and experiential knowledge required for individualized patient care is not recognized by the dominant paradigm as scientific, and hence as valid knowledge, and the research methodologies of the social sciences and of medicine which are promoted within the technical rationality paradigm are simply not capable of producing such knowledge.

This chapter has attempted to lay the foundations for a new paradigm of PCR whose aim is to facilitate the generation of personal and experiential knowledge. Because this knowledge is very different from that advocated and produced by traditional scientific research methodologies, the underlying values and philosophy of the two paradigms stand in stark contrast. Some of these differences have already been explored, and are summarized in Table 3.1.

Although the philosophy of PCR might appear to conflict with

Table 3.1   A comparison of the paradigms of technical rationality and PCR

Technical rationality research	Practitioner-centred research
Generates scientific knowledge and theory for practice	Generates personal and experiential knowledge from practice
Maintains a clear distinction between the researcher and the practitioner	Sees no distinction between researcher and practitioner
Is research into others	Is research into ourselves
Seeks to overcome subjectivity	Seeks to embrace subjectivity
Seeks objectivity and the scientific perspective	Seeks 'prejudice' and the practice perspective
Aims for discovery of knowledge	Aims for creation of knowledge and the development of practice
Appeals to scientific method as the basis for clinical decisions	Appeals to professional judgement as the basis for clinical decisions
Seeks to be rigorous	Seeks to be systematic
Aims for statistical generalizability	Aims for analytical generalizability
Employs random sampling methods	Employs theoretical sampling methods

technical rationality, it is not intended that it should be viewed as a replacement. Rather, the two paradigms have different aims and produce different types of knowledge for different purposes, and in order to make professional judgements of the kind described in Part One of this book, the nurse requires personal, experiential *and* generalizable scientific knowledge.

However, before you consider conducting PCR, it must be pointed out that the nursing establishment is very much opposed to this particular challenge to the dominant paradigm. The Department of

Health Taskforce on the Strategy for Research in Nursing, Midwifery and Health Visiting stated that 'not ... all practitioners should be carrying out research as part of their professional role or their professional development' and that 'the proliferation of inadequately supervised, small-scale projects should be curbed' (Department of Health, 1993). The International Council of Nurses (1996) added that 'significant advances in knowledge rarely result in any field from small-scale individual projects', a rather myopic view since this is precisely how many innovations in the 'hard' sciences have come about.

It is not surprising, therefore, that the initiation by the nurse of small-scale projects to verify her own knowledge-base rarely takes place, and that PCR is a little-explored concept in comparison to the vast amount written about traditional scientific research. This chapter has identified three methodologies for conducting research into our own practice. Some are already well-established ways of doing traditional scientific research, some would probably not be considered by most traditionalists as research at all. Each of these methodologies will now be explored in turn, starting with single-case experimental research.

Notes for Chapter 3

1. It can also be seen from this example that the way the sample is chosen for an analytical generalization is different from the way the sample is chosen for a statistical generalization. For statistical generalizations, where the findings of the research are to be extended to a wider population, it is usual to select a random sample before data collection takes place. In contrast, for analytical generalizations where the findings are used to construct and refine a theory, the sample is generated during the study in response to the emerging data, what Glaser and Strauss (1967) referred to as 'theroetical sampling'.
2. I have categorized nursing research elsewhere (Rolfe, 1996) as a hierarchy of levels. According to that model, reflective research is at level 3 and reflexive research is at level 4. Replicative research is not usually seen as part of a strategy for nursing research, and does not easily fit into the model.
3. It is important that we distinguish between methods and methodologies. As Mills (1959) pointed out, 'methods are the procedures used by men to understand or explain something. Methodology is a study of methods ...'. In other words, methods are our data collection tools, such as questionnaires or interviews, whereas methodologies are the philosophies or organizing frameworks of how those methods are to be employed, such as surveys or phenomenological studies.

4

Single-case experimental research

Background and rationale

Historical development

Single-case experimental research (SCER) was developed by practising psychotherapists and clinical psychologists as a response to the limitations of generalizable research findings for their individual clinical work. It was an attempt to apply the rigor and objectivity of the scientific method to the evaluation of clinical treatments on individual patients by developing an experimental alternative to the randomized controlled clinical trial. Of all the methodologies considered in this book, SCER is the most scientific, and takes its values and design principles from the positivist technical rationality paradigm.

Although developed by clinical psychologists, SCER has its roots in physiology and human learning, particularly in the work of Paul Broca in the 1860s and Hermann Ebinghaus 20 years later. Broca was a physiologist who began to map the functions of the brain by careful examination of brain-damaged patients followed on their death by autopsy. In this way, he managed to employ a single-case methodology to match clinical signs and symptoms with physical damage in order to discover, for example, the speech centre of the brain. Ebinghaus was one of the pioneers of the new discipline of psychology, and is mainly remembered for the discovery of the retention curve in the field of human learning research, which he developed by using himself as the subject of his single-case experiments.

Further developments in the use of single cases in clinical psychology arose out of the case study method employed by Breuer and Freud at the end of the nineteenth century, and later by behavioural psychologists such as Watson. For example, Breuer demonstrated in the case of 'Anna O' how the symptoms of hysteria could be eliminated one at a time by systematically tracing them back to their origins, and Watson employed the case of 'Little Albert' to show how phobic reactions could be systematically extinguished by operant conditioning.

By the 1950s, many clinical psychologists were seriously concerned about the problems related to the generalizability of scientific research, and the clinical case study was developed in two ways. First, many clinical researchers turned to naturalistic studies which involved 'live, unaltered, minimally controlled, unmanipulated "natural" psychotherapy sequences – so-called experiments of nature' (Kiesler, 1971). This approach to case-study research was particularly appealing because it did not interfere with the day-to-day clinical work of the practitioner, and was typified by multiple measures of a wide range of patient and therapist variables.

In the 1960s a second way of doing clinical case study was developed. This was through process research, which was concerned with what went on between the therapist and the patient *during* therapy rather than on the outcome of the therapeutic process. Whilst clearly an important focus of enquiry, it lead to 'an unfortunate distinction between process and outcome studies' in which:

> process research collected data on patient changes at one or more points during the course of therapy, usually without regard for outcome, while outcome research was concerned only with pre-post measures outside of the therapeutic situation.
>
> (Barlow and Hersen, 1984)

Modern-day single-case experimental research was first proposed in the 1970s by the clinical psychologists Bergin and Strupp. Dissatisfied with naturalistic studies as lacking in rigor, and process research as failing to address the real issues of psychotherapy, they suggested the individual case study and the quasi-experimental approach as 'the primary strategies which will move us forward in our understanding of the mechanisms of change at this point' (Bergin and Strupp, 1970). These strategies were finally combined in the work of Barlow and Hersen (1973) and Leitenberg (1973), and later by Bromley (1986), and formulated into a compelling argument against large group research.

Research questions

We have already seen that SCER is useful to the practitioner–

researcher for a number of reasons. Because it is an effective way of isolating important treatment variables, it can be employed for the situational verification of published research in the practitioner's own practice setting, it can be used to test hypotheses based on the practitioner's own personal and experiential knowledge, and it can be used to extend personal and scientific theories to other practice settings and patient groups through naturalistic and analytical generalizations. In its multiple baseline form, it can even be employed as a problem-solving approach by comparing the effectiveness of a number of clinical treatments on a previously intractable problem.

Not surprisingly, then, SCER lends itself to a number of the different types of research question identified in the previous chapter. In terms of the *form*, SCER is concerned mainly with descriptive questions, questions which attempt to understand or describe a situation by establishing relationships between two variables. Indeed, as we have seen, the isolation of all the extraneous variables, leaving only those relevant to the study, is one of the strong points of this particular approach.

It might appear at first sight that SCER is also useful for answering developmental questions, questions which attempt to improve the situation being studied. However, although SCER clearly has an action component in as much as we are measuring the effectiveness of a particular clinical intervention, the variables under investigation are carefully controlled. This method therefore lacks the reflexivity required to modify and re-evaluate treatment approaches which do not appear to be successful while the research is in progress. Whilst SCER is useful for evaluating clinical change, it is of limited use in developing and improving practice.

Turning next to the *focus*, most questions in SCER are practice-based and focus on the practitioner's clinical work; indeed, that is precisely the reason for the development of this particular methodology. Questions can also be organizational, however, and focus on care management issues such as the organization of care, time or resources.

Finally, the *subject* of the questions can either be personal, relating to the practitioner herself, or environmental, relating to her working environment. In the typology employed in the previous chapter, SCER is therefore able to address four kinds of questions, as shown in Figure 4.1

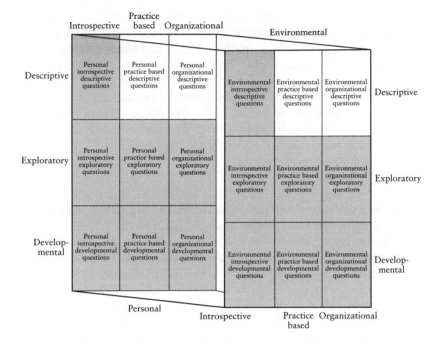

Figure 4.1   *Single-case experimental research questions.*

Methodology and research design

As Peck (1989) pointed out, there are no standard procedures for SCER, but rather:

> a series of experimental manipulations all designed to demonstrate a functional relationship between two variables, such as treatment and outcome. Typically, this involves systematically altering one variable, and observing its effects on the other.

The attraction of this approach for the practitioner–researcher is in the degree of autonomy she can exercise over the research process in order to accommodate it into her everyday practice. As Peck continued, 'as long as the basic logic is followed, it is entirely up to the clinical researcher to use whatever design he feels to be appropriate'.

We can nevertheless identify three broad approaches to single-case experimental research: ABAB designs, multiple baseline designs and alternating treatment designs. ABAB designs involve repeatedly applying and withdrawing a single treatment regimen in order to evaluate its effectiveness, whereas multiple baseline designs allow for several clinical problems or patients to be subjected to the same treatment regimen, and alternating treatment designs enable several interventions to be compared on a single patient. All of these basic types include within them a large number of variations, but in each type, the characteristic of SCER is the systematic way in which the treatment is evaluated by controlling for extraneous variables. All three of these strategies will now be examined in depth.

ABAB designs

There are a number of variations on the ABAB design of measurement and treatment within a single case. As Morley (1989) noted, 'the central feature of experimentation is the comparison of two or more conditions. In single case research these comparisons are made within an individual'. In its simplest form, the comparison is between the measure of a particular variable before and after treatment. This is usually known as the AB design, where A is a baseline measure on, say, a depression rating scale before counselling, and B is the measure on the same rating scale after counselling. The logic of the design is that any improvement between A and B represents the effect of the treatment (Figure 4.2).

Peck (1989) pointed out, however, that this design has a number of obvious weaknesses, the greatest of which is the fact that the relationship between treatment and improvement in the condition has only been demonstrated on one occasion, and 'there could be many other factors to account for the change in the patient's condition, apart from the initiation of treatment'. It is possible in this case that the remission was spontaneous, and that scores on the depression rating scale would have improved anyway, whether or not counselling was provided, or that the treatment coincided with a change in some other significant variable.

A similar design, known as ABA, overcomes this basic weakness by including a further phase of no treatment following the treatment phase (Figure 4.3). For example, a baseline measure of depression is taken and the counselling intervention is introduced, during which time we would expect the rating scores to go down. The treatment is then withdrawn, and if the scores go up again, then 'one can conclude with a high degree of certainty that the treatment variable is the agent responsible for observed changes in the target behaviour' (Barlow and Hersen, 1984).

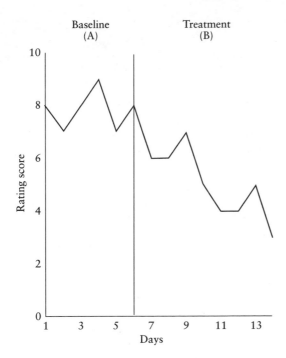

Figure 4.2   *A simple AB design.*

However, the major flaw in the ABA method is not a logical one but an ethical one. Thus:

> On an ethical and moral basis it certainly behooves the experimenter-clinician to continue some form of treatment to its ultimate conclusion subsequent to the research aspects of the case. A further design, known as the A-B-A-B design, meets this criticism as the study ends on the B or treatment phase.
>
> (Barlow and Hersen, 1973)

Thus, while the AB and the ABA designs might be of use where time factors or clinical aspects of the case do not permit an extended research programme, the full ABAB design should usually be the first choice.

ABAB design (Figure 4.4) in which the treatment is given, withdrawn and then given again, is in effect a replication, and as such, it strengthens the validity of the findings. As Sapsford and Abbott (1992) observed:

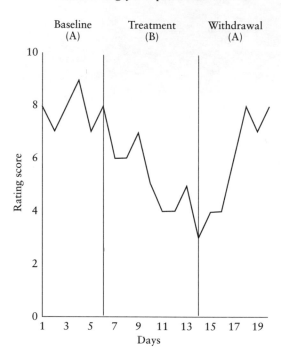

Figure 4.3   *ABA withdrawal design.*

if the probability of a chance result is low when you do the research once, then the chances multiply when you do it twice and get the same result. The chance of drawing the King of Spades from the pack is 1 in 52. The chances of doing so twice are 1 in $52 \times 52 = 2704$ – vanishingly small.

In fact, Sapsford and Abbott are not entirely correct in their statistical analysis, since it is possible that the chance result might be due to different circumstances in each case. Nevertheless, the principle still holds that the strength of the findings is improved if those findings can be demonstrated on more than one occasion. Furthermore, the ABAB design is not limited to a single replication, but can continue as many times as necessary, for example, ABABABAB ...

Before exploring the problems associated with ABAB designs, I shall briefly examine one more approach, namely the BAB design. As its name suggests, BAB design begins with treatment, followed by withdrawal, and then the reinstatement of the treatment. Although not as powerful as the ABAB design, it is useful for evaluating the

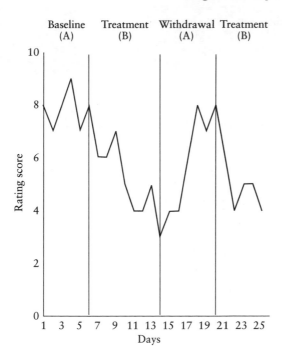

Figure 4.4 *ABAB design.*

effects of treatment procedures which are already under way, and where it is not possible to obtain baseline measures. With an effective treatment, we would expect changes when the treatment is withdrawn, followed by a reversal of those changes when it is reintroduced (Figure 4.5).

Problems with ABAB designs

As we might expect, there are a number of problems associated with the implementation of ABAB single-case experimental research in the practice setting. First, there is the ethical dilemma of withdrawing a treatment which appears to be effective, although of course we cannot be certain of its effectiveness until after we have withdrawn it. Nevertheless, by the second or third time around the ABAB cycle, the evidence for its efficacy is certainly building up. Secondly, it might be necessary to continue observations or measurements when the practitioner–researcher is off duty, and that requires the cooperation

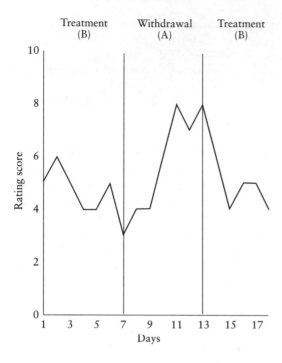

Figure 4.5   *BAB design.*

of colleagues, which in turn might introduce inter-rater reliability problems. Thirdly, the patient might well be discharged before the research programme is completed, particularly if he appears to respond to the initial treatment intervention. Fourthly, the effects of the intervention might take a long time to wear off, or they might not be reversible at all, as with the earlier example of telling a patient that he is dying: once he has been told, he cannot be 'untold'.

Quite often, then, the practitioner–researcher has to make do with a simple AB design, that is, systematic and regular assessments of the patient before and during treatment, although there are a number of weaknesses associated with this design, as Peck (1989) pointed out:

> if the same systematic approach is to be adopted with many patients with similar problems, the accumulation in knowledge would be extremely valuable, particularly if the data enabled one to relate patient characteristics to outcome.

Thus, by carefully selecting our subjects, it is possible not only to build up experiential knowledge about the effectiveness and applications of particular nursing interventions, but to construct, test and modify nursing theories in a far more precise and accurate way than can be achieved by large group generalizable research.

Multiple baseline designs

As we have seen, it is not always possible or desirable continually to apply and withdraw the treatment, and the practitioner–researcher is often forced to rely on a simple AB design that allows for only a single application. In these cases, we can never be entirely certain that any change in the patient's condition is related to the treatment, although as Peck claimed above, we can to some extent control for this by applying the AB methodology to a number of patients with similar problems. The difficulty, of course, is that we might not always have access to enough patients, and this is where multiple baseline designs can be of use.

In fact, Peck's suggestion of applying the same methodology to different patients is one form of multiple baseline design, known as 'multiple baseline across subjects' design. However, the most common form is multiple baseline across problems, where:

> a number of responses are identified and measured over time to provide baselines against which changes can be evaluated. With these baselines established, the experimenter then applies an experimental variable to one of the behaviors, produces a change in it, and perhaps notes little or no change in the other baselines.
>
> (Baer *et al.*, 1968)

Taking a nursing example, the practitioner–researcher might wish to assess the effectiveness of a new treatment for leg ulcers on a particular patient with a number of ulcers. She would first initiate baseline measurements of the ulcers, and then introduce the treatment to one of them, whilst continuing to take baseline measures of the others. If the treatment is effective, we would expect the ulcer to which the treatment is being applied to respond while the other ulcers show no improvement.

The practitioner–researcher would then apply the treatment to a second ulcer, whilst continuing to treat the first and to take baseline measures of the others. She would continue to apply the new treatment to each in turn in a random sequence until all the ulcers had been treated (Figure 4.6). The strength of this design is first in the replications across a number of problems, and secondly in the varying

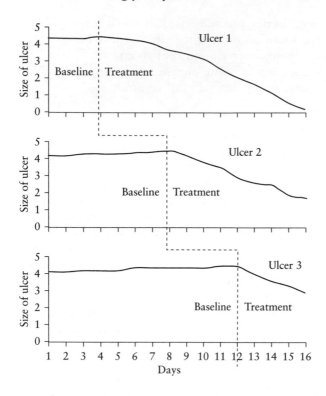

Figure 4.6   *Multiple baseline design.*

lengths of the baselines, which helps to control for other variables which might produce the change, and indeed for 'spontaneous' change. Thus:

> It may be concluded that the treatment has been effective if an improvement is observed in each problem soon after the treatment has been applied; if no improvement is observed, or if one or more of the problems improve before the onset of treatment, then it cannot be concluded that the treatment is responsible for any improvement.
>
> (Peck, 1989)

However, as with ABAB design, multiple baseline designs can only indicate the effectiveness of a treatment in comparison to lack of treatment. If we wish to make comparisons between different treatments in the way that between-group trials are able to do, then we require yet another design.

Alternating treatment designs

We have seen, however, that between-group trials, where one group of patients receives treatment A and a matched group receives treatment B, are prone to intersubject variability which leads to problems in generalizing from the group average to the individual subjects. As Barlow and Hersen (1984) pointed out:

> an ideal solution would be to divide the subject in two and apply two different treatments simultaneously to each identical half of the same individual.

In view of the enormous practical and ethical difficulties involved in dividing our patients into two equal halves, a compromise is required! Such a compromise is the alternating treatment design, which as its name suggests, is 'the rapid alternation of two or more treatments or conditions within a single subject' (Barlow and Hersen, 1984). By rapid, we do not necessarily mean hourly, or even daily, but perhaps that each time a patient is treated, whether it is daily, weekly or monthly, either treatment A or treatment B is given.

Clearly, alternating treatment design can only be employed where the effects of the treatments are of relatively short duration in order to avoid carryover effects. For example, if the two treatments are anti-depressant drugs, there is no point in giving drug B until the effect of drug A has worn off. There might also be a problem with sequential confounding, where the effect of treatment B might be different if given after treatment A than it would have been if given alone. For this reason, the sequence of the interventions is randomized, so rather than proceeding in a simple A-B-A-B-A-B-A-B fashion, we might sequence the interventions as A-B-B-A-B-A-A-B, and so on.

Taking a nursing example, we might wish to compare the effectiveness of two different health education methods on medication compliance. By randomizing methods A and B over a series of eight weekly sessions, a picture might begin to emerge (Figure 4.7). Because we are interested in comparing two interventions rather than in a trend over time, we would not simply connect the data points for weeks 1, 2, 3, and so on, but rather, we would connect all the points representing the effectiveness of intervention A and all the points representing the effectiveness of intervention B. And as Barlow and Hersen (1984) noted:

> If, over time, these two series of data points separated (ie, Treatment B, for example, produced greater improvement than Treatment A), then one could say with some certainty that Treatment B was the most effective.

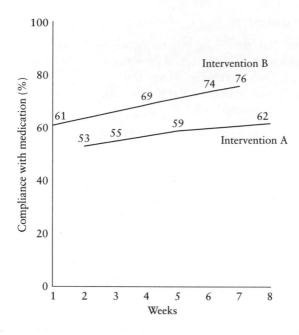

Figure 4.7   *Alternating treatment design.*

They continued: 'Naturally, these results would then need replication on additional clients with the same problem'. If the same trend was noted across several patients, then we would have some empirical justification for continuing to employ method B with other similar patients.

Other design issues

Although a number of SCER designs have been presented as discrete entities, we must beware of taking a 'cookbook' approach. As Morley (1989) emphasized, 'a cardinal feature of single case methods is that experimental designs are flexible – within certain limits – and can be tailored to particular situations'. Rather than adhering slavishly to a fixed design from the book, the practitioner–researcher should adopt what Hayes (1981) referred to as 'an attitude of investigative play' in which the research design is adopted to meet the specific needs of the individual clinical situation.

Probably the most important and least predictable element of SCER design is deciding on the length of the baseline and treatment periods. Unlike most formal research situations, where every element of the design of the study is determined beforehand, decisions about research design in practice-based studies is often made during the research process itself. There are two prime considerations when deciding on the lengths of the different phases: first, the amount of time spent establishing both the baseline and the treatment phases will depend on the emerging data from the study, and secondly, it will depend on the practical clinical considerations of the case.

Starting with the baseline phase, Baer *et al.* (1968) recommended continuing with measurements 'until its stability is clear', or until a predictable pattern emerges. Morley (1989) recommended that the baseline should always be longer than the time in which it is expected that the treatment will take effect: thus, slow-acting treatments require longer baselines than fast-acting ones. However, as Barlow and Hersen (1984) pointed out, this ideal might be overridden by practical clinical considerations, such as an impending discharge or the ethical implications of continuing to withhold a treatment which appears to be effective. Furthermore, such decisions are often not the nurse's to make, and she must work within medically set constraints. Nevertheless, the flexibility of the methodology allows for most problems of this nature to be worked around.

When deciding on the length of the treatment phase, there are a number of issues to be considered. First, it depends on the stability of the baseline. Morley (1989) recommended that in situations where there is considerable variability in the baseline measure, treatment should continue for at least as long as the baseline in order to determine whether or not the pattern has changed. In contrast, if the baseline is stable and the treatment effect is powerful, then a short treatment phase is all that is required to demonstrate an effect.

The treatment phase might also be cut short for clinical reasons, for example, if the intervention is counter-therapeutic, but in such cases it is always advisable to try to determine the reason for the effect, since it might well be transient. For example, in counselling a patient who has recently been given some bad news, he might display anger or acute distress and appear to get worse before starting to come to terms with the news, and this should clearly be taken into account when assessing the therapeutic value of the intervention.

Another reason for withdrawing treatments is if they appear not to be working, but again we must remember that there might be a delay before an intervention begins to take effects, and we should therefore not be too hasty in discontinuing it. As Morley (1989) cautioned, 'investigators should guard against *reactive withdrawal* of treatments'.

In addition to length of treatment, the practitioner–researcher might also wish to vary the type of treatment during the study in response to feedback from the patient. This is, of course, counter to standard scientific procedure, where the treatment variable is applied in a consistent manner, and should be done cautiously. However, conducted in a methodical way, this procedure allows SCER to become reflexive and to bring about improvements in care directly rather than simply measuring and comparing different clinical interventions. Now look at the Reflective Break on page 117.

Data collection methods

Clearly, in order to be able to make direct A-B comparisons, the data collected in single-case experimental research must be quantitative. Furthermore, since analyses are usually made visually by comparing graphs, the data must be either interval or ratio. In other words, the interval between scores of, say, 1 and 2 on a depression rating scale must be the same as the difference between scores of 2 and 3 in order that accurate and meaningful conclusions can be drawn.

However, within these constraints, a wide range of established methods can be used, although if the aim is to test the findings of a previous study in our own clinical areas, then the data collection methods of the original study should be employed as far as possible. It is beyond the scope of this book, however, to describe quantitative research data collection methods, which can be found in almost any nursing or social science research text. The aim here is rather to provide a broad outline of the wide range of variables for which it is appropriate to employ SCER methodology.

Physiological measures

The aim of all data collection methods in SCER methodology is to translate the variables we want to compare into numbers which can be plotted onto a graph. The variables which lend themselves most readily to this treatment are physiological states, many of which can be converted directly into quantitative data. For example, if we wish to compare the size of a leg ulcer before and after treatment, we can take direct measurements by using a tape measure, and these can be plotted on a graph without any intervening and possibly distorting transitions.

REFLECTIVE BREAK

VERIFYING SCIENTIFIC RESEARCH

Think of a piece of scientific clinical research that you have implemented (or are thinking of implementing) in your practice. Design a SCER to verify the findings in your own practice area. Give as much detail as you are able.

Why is this the most appropriate SCER design for your project?

What problems do you foresee in carrying it out?

However, as soon as we move away from direct measurements of this kind, we have to be aware that what we are measuring is not the variable itself, but a more or less artificial representation of it. In some cases, these indirect measures might retain much of the validity and reliability of direct measures. For example, we might wish to measure the size of internal tumours from ultrasound screens, or temperature from the expansion of mercury in a glass tube. In either case, the technology employed to translate the physiological state into a numerical measure is fairly valid and reliable.

However, the variables we wish to study might require a rather less direct approach to measurement; we might, for example, want to compare stress levels before and after a counselling intervention. In this case, we could measure galvanomic skin resistance, which has been associated with stress. However, it is important to be aware that we are not measuring stress itself, but a numerical representation of a physiological state which is thought to be to some extent related to stress. This is an important consideration in quantitative research which, as we shall see, has a direct bearing on the construct validity of the study. The danger is that it is very easy to become so engrossed in a discussion of the data that we forget exactly what it is that we are discussing, and that somewhere in the process we might forget that we are actually comparing measurements of skin resistance and start talking as though we are directly measuring levels of stress.

Measures can be taken either by the subject himself, as in the case of a 'pain thermometer' where he is asked to rate his pain on a scale of, say, one to ten, or by the researcher, who might attempt to rate a patient's depression by an assessment of his behaviour. Once again, this is an important consideration that might affect the validity and reliability of the study.

On the one hand, the subject has a more direct access to his own internal states than does the researcher, who can only infer them from the subject's behaviour. But on the other hand, those very states might well affect the reliability of his reporting. For example, the subject can assess his own level of depression directly. However, one of the features of depression is that we tend to see situations as worse than they really are, and so a depressed subject might well overestimate the depth of his own depression.

Measures of attitude and opinion

There are a large number of validated quantitative measures of attitudes and opinions, and as with physiological instruments, these range from more or less direct to very indirect measures. The most direct measures of attitudes and opinions are simple satisfaction ratings, where, for example, the patient might be asked to rate his satisfaction of a service on a scale of nought to ten.

Rather less direct are psychological self-completion instruments such as the Likert scale for measuring attitudes, and the growing selection of quality of life scales. The most indirect measures of attitudes and opinions are those instruments which are completed by the researcher rather than by the subject, where typically the attitude is inferred by the former from the behaviour of the latter.

Measures of behaviour

The usual method for collecting quantitative data about behaviour is through non-participant observation. The kinds of data collected by this method can range from simple and direct counts of the duration or frequency of certain behaviours, for example, the length of nurse–patient interactions or the number of times a nurse touches a patient during the interaction, through to numerical assessments of the quality of the interaction, for example, by the use of dementia care mapping (Kitwood and Bredin, 1994). As well as the nurse-researcher carrying out the rating, we might also ask the patient, say, to rate the frequency or quality of nurses' behaviours.

Measures of knowledge

Finally, we might wish to measure knowledge, for example, in order to assess the effectiveness of a health education programme. Again, this can be done more or less directly by employing multiple choice tests, or indirectly through the use of open-ended questions which are scored by the researcher.

Validity and reliability

The validity and reliability of a study are issues which apply both to the methodology or study design and to the data collection methods employed within that methodology. With single-case experimental research, both the methodology and the methods are well established, and only a cursory discussion is required.

Validity is usually considered as two separate issues: internal and external validity. The external validity refers to the extent to which the findings from a study can be generalized to wider populations, and has been discussed at some length earlier in Part Two.

The internal validity is the extent to which the data collection instruments measure what they claim to measure. A metre rule is valid if it actually measures in centimetres and metres, rather than, say, in feet and inches; a depression inventory is valid if it measures depression rather than anxiety. In the case of fairly direct measures such as leg ulcer size, the issue of internal validity is clear cut; there can be little disagreement that when we put a tape measure across a leg ulcer, we are measuring what we claim to be measuring, that is, the diameter of the ulcer.

In less direct cases, there might be some dissention. When we take a reading from a thermometer which has been placed in the mouth of a patient, it might on first glance appear that we are measuring his temperature, but what we are actually measuring is the expansion of a column of mercury in a glass tube. Fortunately, there is a well-established correlation between temperature and the expansion of mercury, and we can therefore claim that our instrument has a high internal validity: we wish to measure the temperature of our patient, and that is what we are doing, albeit indirectly.

With more indirect measures, such as attitude scales, we have to be very aware of the issue of internal validity. Attitudes are internal psychological constructs, and it is impossible to gain direct access to them in the same way that we can gain access to a leg ulcer. What we are measuring when we administer a Likert scale is not the subject's internal mental state, but his expressed level of agreement with a number of written statements which relate to that internal state.

By assigning a numerical score to a subject's level of agreement with the statement that smoking is a bad habit, we must not be seduced into thinking that we have necessarily measured his attitude towards smoking. Most established attitude scales have been tested for validity, and it is advisable wherever possible to employ a previously validated tool when conducting SCER.

The reliability of an instrument refers to its accuracy: a metre rule is reliable if it really is a metre long; a depression inventory is reliable if it correlates with actual levels of depression. An instrument can be reliable but not valid, as for example when we try to measure in centimetres with an accurate foot rule. It can also be valid but not reliable, as in the case of measuring in centimetres with an inaccurate metre rule. Most established instruments will have been tested for reliability.

There are several types of reliability apart from straightforward accuracy, two of which will be briefly discussed here. The first, and probably the most important for SCER, is test-retest reliability. This refers to the consistency with which an instrument measures over time. For example, a metre rule which expanded significantly in the heat might give different readings from day to day, depending on the temperature, and would therefore have low test-retest reliability.

Test-retest reliability is clearly an important issue when we are making comparisons over time. If we wish to determine whether a particular treatment reduces the size of leg ulcers, we must be sure that our instrument is actually recording the lessening diameter of the ulcer rather than the temperature of the room in which the measurements are being made.

There are two ways to maximize test-retest reliability. The first is to check that the instrument has a high reliability coefficient, and the second is to ensure that the conditions under which it is administered are as similar as possible on each occasion. Test-retest reliability is rarely 100 per cent, but we must ensure that the magnitude of change attributed to unreliability is of a far lesser order than the magnitude of the change we are trying to measure in our experiment. For example, an expansion of 1 mm in our ruler is acceptable if we are measuring something that is 1 m long, but not if we are measuring something that is only 2 or 3 mm.

The other form of reliability to be briefly discussed here is inter-rater reliability, which is the error induced by asking different people to measure the same variable. Clearly, in much single-case experimental research this is not a problem, since the practitioner–researcher will be doing all the data collection herself. It becomes an issue, however, where the researcher employs her colleagues to collect data on her days off, or when more than one subject is completing self-rating scales. Inter-rater reliability can never be eliminated, but can be minimized by training the data collectors in standardized techniques, and by ensuring that the conditions under which the data are collected are as uniform as possible.

Data analysis

Kazdin (1984) pointed out that data analysis consists of methods that are used to draw conclusions about therapeutic change, and that in SCER, two criteria are usually invoked to evaluate that change. First, and most importantly, there is the therapeutic criterion, which is

concerned with whether the effects of the intervention are therapeutically significant. Thus:

> even if ... change is reliably and clearly related to the experimental
> intervention, the change may not be of clinical or applied significance.
> To achieve the therapeutic criterion, the intervention needs to make an
> important change in the client's everyday functioning.
>
> (Kazdin, 1984)

For example, the rating of a patient on a depression scale might fall
over time by what appears to be a significant amount, and yet the
patient might still be suicidal. It is only by observing and working
with the patient that we can accurately assess whether the intervention has any clinical worth. The advantage that the practitioner–
researcher has over her non-practising research colleagues is that she
is ideally placed to evaluate the clinical significance of any change that
occurs during or after her research. Other methods suggested by
Kazdin for evaluating the therapeutic criterion include comparing the
patient with 'normal' or healthy people, and by asking various people
such as the patient, his relatives or experts to evaluate the magnitude
of the change.

Secondly, there is the experimental criterion, which refers to an
evaluation of the experimental data themselves. As Kazdin (1984)
pointed out:

> The experimental criterion is based on a comparison ... under different
> conditions, usually during intervention and nonintervention (baseline)
> phases. To the extent that performance reliably varies under these
> separate conditions, the experimental criterion has been met.

Assuming that the first criterion of therapeutic significance has
been met, the experimental criterion establishes that the therapeutic
change is as a result of the clinical intervention.

The most usual method of evaluating the experimental criterion is
by simple visual examination of a graphic display of the data, as for
example in Figures 4.2–4.7 in this chapter. However, as Kazdin (1984)
noted, 'to those unfamiliar with the method, visual inspection seems
to be completely subjective and free from specifiable criteria that
guide decision making'. It is therefore imperative that the data are
presented in as unbiased and unambiguous form as possible, and that
great care is taken that any changes over time are neither over- nor
under-emphasized.

The most common way that data are distorted is in the scaling of
the axes. Consider the two graphs in Figure 4.8: both display the same

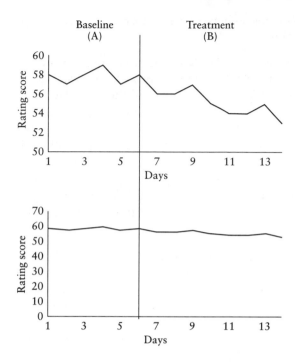

Figure 4.8 *Distortions due to Y axis scaling.*

information, but the effect of treatment in the first graph appears to be much greater than in the second, due to the different ways that the Y (vertical) axis has been scaled.

The danger with the top graph is that the effect of the treatment, represented by a drop in depression rating scores from 58 to 53, might be overestimated, whereas the danger with the bottom graph is that it might be overlooked. The correct scaling depends largely on the clinical judgement of the practitioner–researcher as to the true clinical significance of a drop in depression rating scores from 58 to 53, as well as an assessment as to whether the rating of 53 represents a score in the normal range for the population.

Kazdin (1984) argued that visual inspection should be supplemented by statistical analysis, but as Peck (1989) observed:

> Unfortunately, for technical statistical reasons, the data from the simplest of experimental design (e.g. AB designs) require the most complex of statistical procedures for analysis (e.g.transfer function

analysis). Such methods require sophisticated computer facilities, and a large number of observations, probably over 50.

Fortunately, he claimed, the effects we are seeking are usually quite clear cut, such that 'if statistical analysis is needed to tease out an effect, the effect cannot be of large magnitude in the first place, and may therefore be irrelevant for practical clinical purposes'.

Baer (1977) made a similar point, arguing that a reliance on statistical analysis could result in accepting findings which have statistical but not clinical significance, and Morley (1989) added:

> visual analysis of the data will ensure that type I errors are minimised (i.e. concluding that an effect is present when it is not) but there is a corresponding increase in the likelihood of type II errors (failing to detect an effect when it is present).

As Peck noted above, statistical analysis of SCER data tends to be very complex, and is beyond the scope of this book. The interested reader is therefore referred to Kazdin (1984) for a very thorough review of the subject. However, we have seen that it is generally regarded as being of limited use, and careful graphical presentation of the data is usually quite sufficient.

Summary

Single-case experimental research as a practitioner-centred methodology has been borrowed without modification from psychotherapy research, where it is employed to explore the effectiveness of therapeutic interventions. It is suitable for answering a range of descriptive questions, that is, questions which attempt to understand or describe situations by establishing relationships between two or more variables. As part of a broader strategy of practitioner-centred research, SCER has a number of uses:

- To verify published scientific research in the practitioner–researcher's own clinical area.
- To verify the practitioner–researcher's own personal and experiential knowledge.
- To build and develop practice-based theories.
- To extend personal and scientific knowledge and theories to other practice settings and other patient groups.
- To compare the effectiveness of several clinical interventions.

SCER is scientific and methodical, and involves the systematic manipulation of one variable in order to observe its effect on a second variable. However, within certain constraints it is also very flexible and versatile, and is thus well suited to practitioner-centred research.

There are three broad approaches to designing single-case experimental research studies:

- ABAB designs, where a treatment is repeatedly applied to and withdrawn from a single patient.
- Multiple baseline designs, where the same treatment is applied to a number of patients or to a number of similar problems experienced by the same patient.
- Alternating treatment designs where two or more treatments are applied to the same patient in random order.

Data collection can be achieved by using any quantitative instrument which is capable of generating interval or ratio data, and can include physiological measures, measures of attitude and opinion, measures of behaviour and measures of knowledge. The validity and reliability of the methodology is dependent on the validity and reliability of these individual instruments.

Data analysis is usually carried out by visual inspection and comparison of graphical representations of the data, but care must be taken to ensure that any changes observed are therapeutically significant, and this requires the practitioner–researcher to draw on her own professional judgement. Statistical analysis can be employed, but it tends to be very complex and is of dubious value.

REFLECTIVE BREAK

DESIGNING A SCER PROJECT

Turn back to the personal organizational descriptive question that you formulated in the Reflective Break on page 93. Outline a single-case experiment to answer that question under the following headings:

Problem to be addressed (e.g. what is the problem for *you* in *your* practice?)

Personal interest and prejudice in the problem

Research question (from the Reflective Break on page 93)

Research design (e.g. AB, ABAB, multiple baseline, etc.). Include issues such as length of baseline and treatment phases.

Why is this design most appropriate for your research?

Data collection methods

Ethical and practical constraints

Expected outcomes

5

Reflective case-study research

Background and rationale

Historical development

Case-study research derives from two separate and distinct traditions, the first being psychology and the second being sociology. Its psychological roots are shared with single-case experimental research, and derive from clinical psychologists such as Freud, Breuer and Watson in the late nineteenth and early twentieth century, who employed case histories to illustrate particular treatment methods on individual patients. The sociological roots of case-study research derive from anthropology and the work of pioneers such as Malinowski, Radcliffe-Brown and Evans-Pritchard, who studied whole societies in their natural settings rather than individuals in controlled clinical situations.

The two strands were to some extent brought together by the sociologists of the Chicago School of Ethnography in the 1950s. These ethnographers lived and worked with such diverse groups as homeless men, street gangs, delinquents and dance-hall girls, often singling out particular group members for more detailed study. More recently, researchers from several other disciplines have developed single-case research further, most noticeably in education, where the traditional ethnographic methods of participant observation and interviews have been supplemented by non-participant observation, often using structured instruments, and by questionnaires.

Recently, however, case-study research appears to have fallen from favour, particularly with sociologists, and Yin (1994) has noted that most social science texts no longer consider the case study as a formal research strategy at all. Rather, it is viewed either as the exploratory stage of some larger research study or else it is confused with ethnography or participant observation. Yin further pointed out that, if considered at all, it is taken to be a data collection technique rather than a fully fledged research methodology, or as he described it, a research strategy. In fact, Yin has probably done more than anyone to pull all the threads of case study research together, and is largely responsible for its recent revival.

Definitions

Definitions of case-study research are diverse, often rather vague, and tend to vary from discipline to discipline. Sociologists, for example, rarely use the term 'case study' at all, and usually talk of ethnography, fieldwork or social anthropology, in which the main method is participant observation. As we have already seen, some educationalists have attempted to import ethnographic methods into the study of classroom situations, with Cohen and Manion (1985) claiming that 'at the heart of every case study lies a *method of observation*' (their emphasis). Other educationalists have taken a far broader view. Adelman *et al.* (1976) defined a case study as 'an umbrella term for a family of research methods having in common the decision to focus an inquiry round an instance', whereas Nisbet and Watt (1979) described it merely as 'a systematic investigation of a specific instance'.

Good and Watts (1989), as psychiatrists, were concerned with individual clinical cases rather than classroom groups, but made the similar point that case-study research is distinguished by its theoretical purpose and methodological rigor, and that its aim is usually to add to knowledge or to illuminate. Hartley (1994), on the other hand, writing from the perspective of organizational psychology, saw the focus of case study as organizations or groups within organizations, while Schramm (1971) was concerned with neither individuals, groups nor organizations. He claimed that:

> the essence of a case study, the central tendency among all types of case study, is that it tries to illuminate a decision or set of decisions: why they were taken, how they were implemented, and with what result.

Yin (1994) summarized all these positions, claiming that whilst cases or 'units of analysis' were usually individuals or small groups:

> the "case" can also be some event or entity that is less well defined than a single individual. Case studies have been done about decisions, about programs, about the implementation process, and about organizational change.

Stake (1980) stretched the definition even further, claiming that the case could be any 'bounded system', including 'an institution, a program, a responsibility, a collection, or a population'. Probably the most unstructured definition was offered by Kemmis (1980), who argued that, essentially, a 'case' is whatever happens to be the focus of the case study. Thus:

> the case study worker makes the case a case by carrying out the study. He attempts to transform the situation as an object of perplexity into an object of understanding.

According to this notion of the case, 'case study consists in the imagination of the case and the invention of the study' (Kemmis, 1980).

Yin added the important point that case studies are employed when we wish to investigate a contemporary phenomenon within its real-life context, and he also stressed the need for multiple sources of evidence. He pointed out that case studies can go beyond mere description of a situation to the development and testing of theories. Hakim (1987) expanded this function of case studies further, claiming that:

> At the simplest level they provide descriptive accounts of one or more cases. When used in an intellectually rigorous manner to achieve experimental isolation of selected social factors, they offer the strengths of experimental research within natural settings. In between these two extremes there is an extended range of case studies combining exploratory work, description and the testing out of hunches, hypotheses and ideas in varying combinations.

From these many definitions, we can make some statements about the way that case-study research is usually practised. Case-study research is characterized by bringing to bear a number of different data collection methods to the study of one or more 'cases'. These cases can be individuals, groups, organizations, or even issues or events. The cases are contemporary rather than historical, and are studied in their real-life context rather than under controlled conditions. Finally, case-study research can be simply illuminative or else it can be employed to build or test theory.

Weaknesses of case study research

We can see from this description that case-study research might well be of use to the researcher-practitioner, since it offers a way of generating personal and experiential knowledge in the clinical setting by the practitioner herself. However, before going further, it might be wise to consider some of the identified weaknesses of the case-study approach.

As Yin (1994) claimed, proponents of case-study methodology must refute criticisms of their investigations 'as having insufficient precision, objectivity and rigor', a criticism which he vehemently denied. He also noted that the frequent criticism of case studies as taking too long to conduct largely results from a confusion with ethnography. Nisbet and Watt (1979) added that the weaknesses of case-study methodology include being 'personal and subjective', and as not being generalizable 'except by an intuitive judgement that "this case" is similar to "that case" '. However, from the perspective of the practitioner–researcher, a subjective, personal approach and the ability to generalize from case to case (Stake's 'naturalistic generalizability') are the very qualities that are sought in a research methodology, and what are seen as weaknesses from the perspective of technical rationality turn out to be strengths for practitioner-centred research.

However, there is a more serious criticism which must be considered. The focus of traditional case-study research is on an external 'case', whether an individual, a group or an event, and the aim of the researcher has always been to minimize her impact on the person or event being studied. This approach is referred to as naturalism (May, 1993), which emphasizes that 'the social world should be studied in its "natural state", undisturbed by the researcher' (Hammersley and Atkinson, 1983). For example, in studying classroom interactions, the aim of the non-participant observer is to blend into the background so that she can retain a degree of objectivity and will not influence the interactions she is studying.

Even with participant observation studies, which might adopt an overt position of subjectivity, there still remains the problem of the Hawthorne effect, that the findings of the study are contaminated simply by the presence of the researcher. The mere fact that I am part of the group which I am researching will have an affect on the behaviour of that group, even if I say nothing and make no attempt to influence it in any way. Thus, Burgess (1984) warned of 'the possibility of researchers modifying and influencing the research context as well as being influenced by it themselves', whilst Janes (1961) posed the question: 'how does the community role of the investigator affect statements made by local respondents?'.

Yin (1994) referred to this indirect influence as the problem of reflexivity, that the 'event may proceed differently because it is being observed', echoing Becker's (1958) question: 'to what degree is the informant's statement the same one he might give ... in the absence of the observer?'. Yin also noted the problem of the researcher *directly* influencing the situation she is studying, where, as a group member, she might 'have to assume positions or advocacy roles contrary to the interests of good scientific practices'. Even in the course of simply collecting data, the researcher might exert an influence by asking questions and raising issues which would otherwise not have been raised. The presence of the researcher therefore has both a direct and an indirect influence on the situation she is there to study.

Reflexivity and reflective case-study research

For traditional case-study research, this is indeed a problem, since the aim is to understand or theorize about individuals or groups from their own perspectives and in their natural settings, and to do so in a way that is acceptable to the scientific community. However, as soon as a researcher moves in, the setting is no longer natural. The difficulty, particularly for the participant observer, is therefore to become accepted as part of the group she is studying in order to understand it fully, but at the same time not to influence the group's behaviour either directly or indirectly.

However, although this is a serious problem for traditional case-study methodology, it will be recalled that the focus of PCR is not on some external person or event, but on the practitioner herself and her own practice. It therefore embraces the very reflexivity that Yin rejected, since the aim of PCR is *precisely* to study the effect of the researcher–practitioner on her own clinical practice. The researcher–practitioner is therefore a participant observer of her own clinical work, and it is impossible to separate the roles of observer and observed as it is in the traditional case-study methodology.

Now consider how the participant observer traditionally collects her data. As Becker (1958) noted:

> The participant observer gathers data by participating in the daily life of the group or organization he studies. He watches the people he is studying to see what situations they ordinarily meet and how they behave in them. He enters into conversation with some or all of the participants in these situations and discovers their interpretations of the events he has observed.

Hammersley and Atkinson (1983) pointed out the limitations of memory, and that the data need to be written up as fieldnotes immediately following the period of observation: 'when to write notes? In principle, one should aim to make notes as soon as possible after the observed action that is to be noted'.

And here is Burgess (1984) describing how he kept his fieldnotes of a case study of a school:

> I used diagrams to show the individuals who sat next to each other in meetings and to summarise interactions and conversations between participants. Often these diagrammatic notes were written shortly after the period of observation and provided a summary that could be used later in the day to write up more detailed notes.

But when the case we are studying is ourselves, the fieldnotes will be our recollections about our own behaviours, thoughts and feelings, and like traditional fieldnotes, they should be written up as soon as possible after the event. Thus, when we attempt to collect data by playing the role of participant observer of our own practice, what we are doing is a form of reflection-on-action.

Case-study methodology therefore has the potential for being a very powerful tool for the practitioner–researcher reflectively to explore her own practice, combining the external, quasi-objective data from interviews, document analysis and possibly third-party non-participant observations, with the internal, subjective data from the practitioner–researcher's own reflections-on-action. In order to distinguish case-study research carried out by the practitioner–researcher from the more traditional 'scientific' form, I will refer to it as reflective case-study methodology.

Research questions

Yin (1994) identified a number of different forms of questions that case-study research can address. First, it can answer certain 'what' questions, for example, 'what are the ways of making nursing more effective?'. He referred to these as exploratory questions, and pointed out that although case study research could provide an answer, these questions can, in fact, be addressed by any research methodology.

He also identified a second type of 'what' question such as 'what have been the outcomes of a particular nursing intervention?', which he claimed is actually a form of a 'how much' or a 'how many' question, and which is best answered by a survey, or indeed a single-case experiment as described in the previous chapter. In the terminology employed in this book, these are all descriptive questions, attempts to understand or describe a situation, usually employing quantitative data.

In contrast to these descriptive questions, Yin also identified explanatory questions which deal with operational links needing to be traced over time. These questions usually start with 'how' or 'why', for example, 'why did that intervention produce those outcomes?', and are best answered by case-study research. In the terminology of this book, these are exploratory questions because they explore relationships between variables, and should not be confused with Yin's exploratory questions, which I have referred to as descriptive. To avoid further confusion, I will use my terminology from now on.

With regard to the *form* of the question, then, case-study research can answer some types of descriptive questions, for example 'what are the effects of this nursing intervention?'. These types of questions seek to establish or describe relationships between a number of variables, but they can also be addressed, often more effectively, by other research strategies. However, case-study research is more usefully employed in answering exploratory questions, such as 'why is this nursing intervention more effective than that intervention?', questions which seek to explain or explore relationships, and which usually require qualitative data.

Turning to the *focus* of the questions, we have already seen that traditionally, case studies have been employed to answer questions about individuals, groups, organizations, decisions, the implementation process and organizational change. In the terminology of this book, this includes practice-based questions which focus on the practitioner's clinical work, on her relationship with patients, on the effectiveness of her clinical interventions or on her models and strategies of practice, and also organizational questions which focus on care management issues such as the organization of care, time or resources.

From the perspective of PCR and reflective case-study methodology, however, the focus of the research is not some other practitioner or organization, but the practitioner–researcher herself and her own clinical base. Therefore, although it is relevant to focus the research question on the way that she practises or the way that she organizes her care, a more important focus for the question is an introspective one, which examines the practitioner–researcher herself as a therapeutic agent, and which might be concerned with her personal philosophy of care, her beliefs and attitudes, or her personal qualities, skills, knowledge and expertise. We can see, then, that all three foci can be addressed by reflective case-study research, but that the introspective focus is the most relevant.

Turning finally to the *subject* of the question, case-study research can address both personal questions which relate to practice, and also environmental questions which relate to the working environment of the practitioner–researcher. In the typology of this book, reflective case-study research can be employed to answer 12 kinds of questions, as illustrated in Figure 5.1.

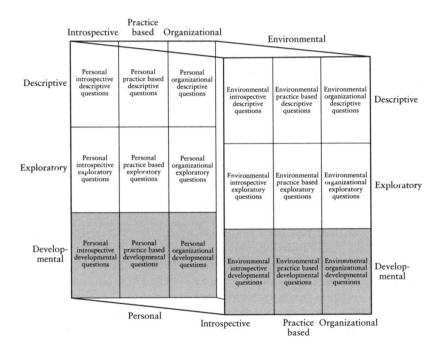

Figure 5.1   *Reflective case-study research questions.*

We can see that there is some overlap between the types of questions addressed by single-case experimental research and those addressed by reflective case-study research, but the questions are answered in very different ways by the different methodologies. In addition, different data collection methods best suit different types of questions, and certain of the questions identified above are more relevant to reflective case-study research than others.

Methodology and research design

The issue of research design in case-study methodology is less clear cut than in SCER. Generally speaking, case studies are characterized by the use of a number of data collection methods to focus on a particular issue or, in Yin's terminology, a proposition. The usual way in which this is achieved is through triangulation, which allows the researcher 'to collect information from multiple sources but aimed at corroborating the same fact or phenomenon' (Yin, 1994). Yin referred to this focusing of several data collection methods on the same issue or case as 'converging lines of enquiry', and claimed that:

> any finding or conclusion in a case study is likely to be much more convincing and accurate if it is based on several different sources of information, following a corroboratory mode.

Within this framework of corroboratory methods, Yin identified five components of a research design that are especially important, namely:

1 a study's questions;
2 its propositions, if any;
3 its unit(s) of analysis;
4 the logic linking the data to the propositions;
5 the criteria for interpreting the findings.

(Yin, 1994)

Of these components, the first has already been considered and the latter two will be explored when we come to look at data analysis. This leaves the issues of deciding on the propositions of the study and choosing the unit(s) of analysis.

We shall first explore the issues involved in identifying the units of analysis of the study, and then go on to discuss the importance of the study propositions or theories. Finally, we shall examine the ways in which both the units of analysis and study propositions exert an influence on the design of the study. We shall contrast single-case and multiple-case studies as ways of building and testing theory, focusing particularly on reflective case-study methodology.

Unit(s) of analysis

The issue of the units of analysis of the study is related to what Yin (1994) called 'the fundamental problem of defining what the "case" is'. As we have seen, in traditional case study research the focus of the case is usually either an individual, such as a particular aspect of a patient's life; a social group, such as the functioning of a ward team; an institution, such as the workings of a community hostel; or an event, such as a clinical emergency or crisis.

Thus, we might choose to study the way that a clinical team in an accident and emergency unit handles breaking bad news to relatives. The 'case' would be a number of instances of breaking bad news, and we could research the case by participant observation, that is, by joining the team in order to study the way they work, by interviews with team members and relatives, and by analysing nursing and medical notes.

However, because the practitioner–researcher is concerned with studying herself and her immediate clinical environment rather than an outside agency, the units of analysis of reflective case-study research are rather different from those of traditional case studies. These differences can be seen in Table 5.1.

Table 5.1   Units of analysis in traditional and reflective case-study research

Focus of the study	Traditional case-study research	Reflective case-study research
Individual case history	Outside person e.g. patient or nurse	Myself and my own practice
Study of a social group	Outside group e.g. clinical team	Clinical team of which I am a member
Study of an institution	Outside institution, e.g. hospital	Hospital in which I work
Study of a specific event	Outside event, e.g. crisis situation	Crisis involving myself

Furthermore, reflective case-study research also includes introspective questions; questions related to the internal world of the practitioner–researcher, for example, her personal philosophy of care, her beliefs and attitudes, or her personal qualities, skills, knowledge and expertise. These are all huge areas, and we must be very careful, particularly when the focus is on ourselves, to delineate clearly the boundaries of the case so that we do not collect a mass of data that is irrelevant to the research question.

An introspective question might be concerned with my own thoughts, feelings and anxieties about how *I* break bad news to relatives. The 'case' in this example would be a number of incidents where I was involved in the breaking of bad news, and the primary tool for exploring the case would be reflection-on-action, the retrospective analysis of my thoughts and feelings about how I break bad news, supplemented by interviews and document analysis.

Study propositions

However, as Yin pointed out, neither the units of analysis nor the research question tell us what we should be studying; the study still requires structure, and that is provided by formulating one or more propositions in the form of hypotheses or a similar theoretical framework. As Hartley (1994) noted:

> without a theoretical framework, a case study may produce fascinating details about life in a particular organization but without any wider significance. Indeed, a case study without the discipline of theory can easily degenerate into a 'story'.

For example, the research question 'why is nursing intervention A more effective than nursing intervention B?' lacks focus and gives no clear indication of where to begin. But as practitioner–researchers, we will have some reason for asking the question, and probably some idea as to its possible answer. We might, for example, try to explain the difference in effectiveness by the proposition that intervention A is more holistic, in which case we would structure our data collection around an exploration of holism. In this way, case-study research can transcend mere description and become a way of formulating and testing theories. We shall see how this is possible later in the chapter.

The key to hypothesis formulation and theory testing is flexibility (Hammersley and Atkinson, 1983),[1] such that 'the strategy and even direction of the research can be changed relatively easily, in line with changing assessments of what is required'. Nevertheless, the researcher usually brings with her a problem or issue from her practice, what Malinowski (1922) referred to as a 'foreshadowed problem'.

The aim is to turn this foreshadowed problem into a set of research questions, although, as Hammersley and Atkinson (1983) pointed out, 'sometimes in this process the original problems are transformed or even completely abandoned in favour of others'. Thus, Hartley (1994) has argued that:

> the initial identification of research questions and theoretical framework will work best where it is tentative – with a recognition that the issues and theory may shift as the framework and concepts are repeatedly examined against the data which are systematically collected.

Nisbet and Watt (1979) made a similar point, that 'in case study, it is possible to preserve a more open approach until the researcher has really begun to "get the feel" of the situation', and suggested that the case study be preceded by an 'open phase' in which the researcher should 'read and observe, but resist the pressure to construct hypotheses or a conceptual framework, and put aside preconceptions'.

This phase, they claimed, is open-ended, can lead to great anxiety and worry, and could last for a very long time. Fortunately the practitioner–researcher has a distinct advantage over the traditional case-study researcher because she is in daily clinical contact with her potential cases, and will embark on her study with some fairly robust questions which will hopefully require little modification.

Single- and multiple-case research

One way of testing a theory is to carry out a number of case studies which gradually eliminate competing theories. However, Yin (1994) has argued that it is also possible to test a theory with a single case, and this brings us to the issue of single- versus multiple-case research. It is important to realize that the number of cases is not necessarily related to the number of individuals being studied. It is possible to conduct a single case study on a social group consisting of many individuals, and it is also possible to conduct a multiple case study of a single person in a variety of situations.

There are two distinct forms of multiple-case research. The first and most common is the comparative case study, where a particular nursing innovation, say, the introduction of primary nursing, is studied over several different sites. Thus, each site would be the subject of an individual case study, and all the individual cases taken together would form a multiple-case design. When applied to PCR, the practitioner–researcher might study the way in which she implements a particular nursing intervention with a number of her patients, each of which would be an individual case, but when taken together would result in a comparative case study.

The more powerful form of multiple-case research is the replication model. Yin (1994) gave the example of case-study research into a rare clinical syndrome where the researcher has access to only three cases. If the three cases do indeed all involve the same syndrome, then the theoretical framework for the study would predict similar outcomes in each case, and the finding of similar outcomes would therefore support the theory. If, on the other hand, dissimilar outcomes were obtained for each of the three cases, then the theory that they each involve the same syndrome would be refuted. This, of course, is Yin's analytical generalization, which was discussed in a previous chapter.

We can see, then, that multiple-case studies can be employed to generate and test theories using very few cases, as long as they are well chosen. Each case must either predict similar results (a literal replication), or produce contrasting results but for predictable reasons (a theoretical replication). As Yin (1994) pointed out:

> The ability to conduct six or ten case studies, arranged effectively within a multiple-case design, is analogous to the ability to conduct six to ten experiments on related topics; a few cases (two or three) would be literal replications, whereas a few other cases (four to six) might be designed to pursue two different patterns of theoretical replications. If all the cases turn out as predicted, these six to ten cases, in the aggregate, would have provided compelling support for the initial set of propositions. If the cases are in some way contradictory, the initial propositions must be revised and retested with another set of cases. Again, this logic is similar to the way scientists deal with contradictory experimental findings.

This form of multiple-case study design provides a very powerful tool for theory building, and is well suited to PCR. For example, it might be that on a particular psychiatric ward, information about medication is sometimes given to patients by the nurse, sometimes by the pharmacist, and sometimes by both, depending on who is available at the time. The practitioner–researcher might wish to test the proposition that, on her ward, information-giving about the effects of medication by the nurse and the pharmacist together results in a gradual improvement in medication compliance in patients suffering from schizophrenia, but that information-giving by either one or the other makes no difference to compliance.

In order to test this theoretical proposition, she might employ a combination of observations, interviews and document analysis to assess increase in compliance in four cases where both the nurse and the pharmacist gave information about the medication, four cases where only the pharmacist gave the information, and four cases where only the nurse gave it.

If she finds that compliance does indeed increase in all the cases when both professionals provide the information but not in the cases when only one or the other is present, then she has strong evidence to support her theory. If, on the other hand, she finds that compliance only increases when the nurse alone gives the information, then her theory will need to be modified and retested.

Yin has argued that it is also possible to test a theory by studying a single 'critical' case. Thus:

> The theory has specified a clear set of propositions as well as the circumstances within which the propositions are believed to be true. To confirm, challenge, or extend the theory, there may exist a single case, meeting all of the conditions for testing the theory. The single case can then be used to determine whether a theory's propositions are correct or whether some alternative set of explanations might be more relevant.

Thus, the practitioner–researcher can test her theory that intervention A is effective with people who show symptom S but not symptoms T, U, V or W by studying one patient who meets these criteria. Hakim (1987) added that we can also disprove a theory by obtaining a positive response to intervention A in a single 'deviant' case who exhibits none of the indicated criteria but all of the contraindicated ones.

Data collection methods

We have seen that traditionally, case-study methodology usually employs several methods of data collection focused on one or more cases, including documentation, archival records, interviews, direct observation and participant observation.[2] A detailed discussion of these methods is beyond the scope of this book, and the interested reader is directed in the first instance to Yin (1994), who provides a very useful discussion of each, with indications for further reading.

We are concerned here, however, with *reflective* case study methodology as a form of practitioner-centred research, and we shall therefore focus our discussion on how the above methods can be of benefit to the nurse who is researching her own practice.

Documentation

Yin pointed out that documentary information is likely to be relevant to every case study topic, and might include:

- Letters, memoranda, and other communiques;
- Agendas, announcements and minutes of meetings, and other written reports of events;
- Administrative documents - proposals, progress reports, and other internal documents;
- Formal studies or evaluations of the same "site" under study;
- Newspaper clippings and other articles appearing in the mass media.

(Yin, 1994)

Burgess (1984) made the distinction: (1) between primary sources such as minutes, letters and diaries, and secondary sources such as transcripts or summaries of primary source material; (2) between public documents such as hospital records and newspaper reports, and private documents such as letters and diaries; and (3) between unsolicited documents which are produced without research in mind, and solicited documents produced at the request of the researcher, such as diaries.

Yin added that the most important use of documentation is to corroborate and augment evidence from other sources, either directly by confirming or challenging previously collected information, or indirectly, for example, by making inferences from the distribution list of a particular set of minutes.

In any case, it should be remembered that written documentation is open to the same charges of bias as other forms of evidence. This bias might be unintentional, since 'no matter what form these various documents take, essential to them all is that they present an individual's subjective view of social life' (Burgess, 1984), or it might be intentional, since written documents 'contain only what someone originally decided to include, and they may omit points which were difficult or inconvenient to include' (Nisbet and Watt, 1979).

Garfinkel (1967) went even further to suggest that records should be regarded as 'contractual' rather than 'actuarial'; that is, they cannot be relied upon as accounts of what actually happened, but only as tokens of the fact that somebody did something to a reasonable standard. Thus, for Garfinkel, the minutes of a meeting are not a reliable guide to what happened in that meeting, but only an indication that the meeting took place and that certain people were present.

However, Hammersley and Atkinson (1983) urged that documents be accorded neither too little nor too much importance: 'like other accounts, they should be read with regard to the context of their production, their intended audience(s), and the author's interests and motives'. They continued with a list of questions that the researcher should ask herself:

How are documents written? How are they read? Who writes them? Who reads them? For what purposes? On what occasions? With what outcomes? What is recorded? What is omitted? What is taken for granted? What does the writer seem to take for granted about the reader(s)? What do readers need to know in order to make sense of them?

(Hammersley and Atkinson, 1983)

All of the above points apply as much to reflective case-study research as to more traditional forms. However, because the documents from which the data are taken will relate to the practitioner–researcher herself, to her work, and to her own clinical area or institution, there are a number of issues which might affect the selection, analysis and presentation of documents in PCR which do not apply to traditional research.

First, there is the issue of access to the documents. As a member of the organization she is studying, the practitioner–researcher will have day-to-day access to much of the relevant documentation, and this can be both an advantage and a disadvantage. The advantage is that the researcher–practitioner is familiar with the range and content of what is available, can freely dip into it, and is not dependent on some other person as a gatekeeper.

However, this free access can itself produce problems. It is easy to forget that permission is still required to use the information for anything other than direct clinical purposes (and of course, PCR will not usually be considered to be a clinical purpose, despite my arguments in this book), and there are all sorts of hidden ethical dilemmas surrounding the use of clinical and managerial documentation which might not be openly addressed if the researcher is not an outside person going through the usual formal channels.

But the fact that the researcher is also a practitioner in the organization where she is conducting her research can also impede access to documentation. There might, for example, be documents of a sensitive organizational nature that would normally be available to detached outside researchers, but which are not considered suitable to be seen by employees of the organization. There might be confidential documents concerning colleagues, or even concerning herself, to which she is denied access, and there might also be medical records which doctors and other health-care professionals would be willing to show to an outside researcher but not to a junior colleague.

Even once access has been negotiated, there will still be problems concerning the selection of documents and of what information from those documents to include in the research study. Because of the practitioner–researcher's status as an employee in the organization she is researching, her employers are in a position to put pressure on her to present the organization in a favourable light in a way that they are unable to do with researchers from outside of the organization.[3] Because many of the documents will relate to her own practice, and to that of her friends and colleagues, there is also the insidious and often unconscious temptation on her part to be selective in the data that are presented in the study.

We can see, then, that although documentation is a useful and important source of data for reflective case-study research, it presents a number of pitfalls that do not exist for the traditional outside researcher, and special care must be taken in the planning stage of the study if documentary evidence is to be included.

Archival records

Yin considered that archival records do not necessarily assume the same importance as other documentation in case-study research, and that their usefulness will vary from study to study. He identified a number of sources of archival material, including:

- Service records, such as those showing the number of clients served over a given period of time;
- Organizational records, such as organizational charts and budgets over a period of time;
- Maps and charts of the geographical characteristics of a place;
- Lists of names and other relevant commodities;
- Survey data, such as census records or data previously collected about a 'site';
- Personal records, such as diaries, calendars, and telephone listings.

(Yin, 1994)

Archival records, like documentation, usually exist in written or computerized form, and most of the considerations and pitfalls identified above apply equally to archive material, although most of it will be of far less personal significance to the practitioner–researcher. In addition, Yin pointed out that archival records are often highly quantitative, 'but numbers alone should not automatically be considered a sign of accuracy'.

This lack of accuracy in statistical records has long been a problem to sociologists, and it prompted the ethnomethodologists such as Cicourel to devise a radical solution:

> For years sociologists have complained about "bad statistics and distorted bureaucratic record-keeping" but have not made the procedures producing the "bad" materials we label "data" a subject of study
>
> (Cicourel, 1976)

Thus, rather than simply accepting the inaccuracy of archival material, we should be exploring how and why it came to be inaccurate. We should remember that:

> most archival records were produced for a specific purpose and a specific audience (other than the case study investigation), and these conditions must be fully appreciated in order to interpret the usefulness of any archival records.
>
> (Yin, 1994)

By taking a hermeneutic approach and looking beyond the data themselves to the underlying reasons for producing them, we are able to open up a whole new area of enquiry which can throw fresh light on the cases being studied. However, because it lacks both a personal and a current focus for the practitioner–researcher, the use of archival records in reflective case-study research is usually in support of other sources of data rather than as a primary research method.

Interviews

Interviews are probably the most widely used form of social research, and are seen by Yin (1994) as one of the most important sources of case-study data. But as Burgess (1984) pointed out, whereas mainstream sociologists usually employ structured interviews:

> few field researchers have followed the structured approach, preferring to use an informal or unstructured or semi-structured style of interviewing which employs a set of themes and topics to form questions in the course of conversation.

This notion of interviews as 'conversations with a purpose' is similar to Yin's concept of 'open ended interviews', in which:

> you can ask key respondents for the facts of a matter as well as for the respondents' opinions about events. In some situations, you may even ask the respondent to propose his or her own insights into certain occurrences and may use such propositions as the basis for further enquiry.
>
> (Yin, 1994)

In fact, Yin considered that the title 'respondent' is inappropriate to such a key role, and suggested instead that he be considered an 'informant', since 'such persons not only provide the case study investigator with insights into a matter but also can suggest sources of corroboratory evidence - and initiate the access to such sources'. Burgess made a similar point, noting that interviews can be used to complement participant observation, helping the researcher to gain access to places and situations that are usually 'closed', and providing data about events that the researcher did not witness.

For example, a key informant in a study of a particular patient might be his primary nurse, who could provide rich and detailed information about the patient and his care, make available particularly important supporting documentation, and facilitate access to the patient himself.

Yin also considered the use of structured interviews and surveys as viable data collection methods for case-study research, particularly for testing already formulated theories and propositions or checking out data collected by other means. However, Hammersley and Atkinson (1983), writing about reflexive ethnography, pointed out that we should not conceive of interviews as either structured or unstructured:

> All interviews, like any other kind of social interaction, are structured by *both* researcher and informant. The important distinction to be made is between standardized and reflexive interviewing. Ethnographers do not decide beforehand the questions they want to ask, though they may enter the interview with a list of issues to be covered. Nor do ethnographers restrict themselves to a single mode of questioning. On different occasions, or at different points in the same interview, the approach may be non-directive or directive, depending on the function that the questioning is intended to serve.

In addition to data collected from formal interview situations, the researcher might also be presented with unsolicited accounts, or what Hammersley and Atkinson (1983) referred to as 'telling the researcher how it is', the aim of which is 'to counteract what it is assumed others have told the researcher, or what are presumed to be his or her likely interpretations of what has been observed'.

Yet another type of interview data for the practitioner–researcher exploring her own practice is data about herself. Sapsford and Abbott (1992) suggested that this can be obtained in two ways. First, the practitioner–researcher can 'interview' herself by keeping a diary which she can then 'study ... as if it were a set of life history interviews with someone else, and analyze it for major themes'. McCarthy

(1994), in a similar vein, wrote of a 'conversation with myself', and Jones (1989), of 'concocting an "imaginary" friend, an interlocutor who would become a springboard for my self-reflection'.

Secondly, the practitioner–researcher can get someone else to interview her, since 'others can push you to clarify ideas which might seem to you self-evidently clear when you write them down' (Sapsford and Abbott, 1992). She therefore has a number of different kinds of interview data at her disposal, including data from herself as well as from solicited and unsolicited interviews with others.

The practitioner–researcher has a number of advantages, as well as several disadvantages, over the outside researcher. The advantages are fairly obvious. First, because she is researching her own practice or clinical area, the practitioner–researcher has a good understanding of the context in which the interview is being conducted, and is able to frame relevant and penetrating questions. Secondly, because the informants are her colleagues, patients and bosses, she has far easier access to them than would an outside researcher. Thirdly, the rapport that is so important, particularly in unstructured interviews, is usually already established before the interview commences.

However, the very factors which facilitate the interviews can also act to distort and disrupt them. The practitioner–researcher is researching her own practice or her own clinical area, and this can lead to a number of difficulties. For example, there is the problem of what Platt (1981) referred to as 'latent identities'. Because the practitioner–researcher will be known to most of the respondents and will have some background knowledge of the issues being researched, 'personal and community knowledge [can be] used as part of the information available to construct a conception of what the interview [was] meant to be about and thus affect what [was] said'. In particular, Platt identified the problem of informants assuming that the researcher would draw on her own background knowledge so that there was no need to spell out the details of what they were saying.

It must also be remembered that the practitioner–researcher is either directly or indirectly the subject of her own interview, and this can cause a number of difficulties. First, there is the problem of the informants telling the researcher what they think she wants to hear. Complements are far easier to give than criticisms, and informants might well find it uncomfortable to be critical of the interviewer, particularly in an unstructured, face-to-face situation. Superiors will probably not find this too difficult, but peers might well have problems, and patients who depend on the practitioner–researcher for their care are likely to have particular difficulties in providing her with honest critical feedback.

As well as experiencing difficulties in obtaining honest responses, the practitioner–researcher might also have problems in being direct and honest herself in the framing of questions to peers and superiors. This is particularly problematical when asking probing questions which challenge their clinical or managerial performance, and in extreme cases, she could find friendships or career prospects being put in jeopardy. This, of course, is equally a problem when the practitioner–researcher is the interviewee rather than the interviewer.

There are also more insidious and possibly unconscious threats to the validity of the data. Just as it is often difficult for informants to provide criticism, so it can be difficult for the practitioner–researcher to hear it. She might well take unconscious steps to avoid acknowledging criticisms of her practice, either by misinterpreting the interview data in a more favourable light, or by structuring the interview and the questions so that the informants only have the opportunity to make positive comments.

There are, of course, a number of problems associated with the use of interviews as part of *any* research methodology, although we have seen that some of these are heightened in practitioner-centred enquiry and some are reduced. These include asking loaded or leading questions, interviewer or respondent bias, poor recall, poor articulation and lack of rapport. A full discussion of these and other issues can be found in any good research text.

However, providing that the practitioner–researcher is aware of the potential problems, there is no reason why both structured and unstructured interviews with herself and her colleagues should not provide a valuable source of data for reflective case-study research, and as Schutz (1994) pointed out:

> The generation of experiential knowledge must require a relationship between researcher and informant which is built on trust, and which will generate familiarity and mutual personal knowledge, and this is more likely to be achieved by a researcher who is previously known to the informant.

Non-participant observation

Nisbet and Watt pointed out that observations can be usefully employed to complement interviews, and that they bring a different perspective to the case study. Observations are direct and enable us to collect data about how people behave in the real world. In contrast, 'interviews reveal how people perceive what happens, not what actually happens' (Nisbet and Watt, 1979). They continued: 'Both the actual events and the perceptions are important data, and so usually you have to combine interview and observation'.

Observations are usually divided into two types: participant or ethnographic observation, and non-participant or direct observation. Some researchers see these methods as diametrically opposed, such that participant observation is an active, subjective immersion in the social setting in order to collect 'natural' qualitative data, and non-participant observation is a passive, objective standing back from the situation in order to collect 'scientific' quantitative data. Other researchers see the methods as essentially similar, and cite the continuum proposed by Gold (1958) which ranges from 'complete participant' to 'complete observer', with a number of intermediate stages along the way. It is to this latter end of the continuum that we shall first turn our attention.

Yin (1994) differentiated between two types of non-participant observation, namely formal data collection activities which usually involve a data collection protocol or structured tool, and informal activities, such as observations of buildings or office furnishings, which can be carried out whilst collecting other data, for example, during an interview. In reflective case study research, informal data collection of this type is usually unnecessary, since the practitioner–researcher will probably be familiar with the setting she is observing.

In fact, the whole issue of formal non-participant data collection techniques in PCR is fraught with difficulties. This is particularly so where the practitioner–researcher is carrying out research into herself or her own clinical team, since she is, by definition, a participant in what she is researching. It is only when she is studying the wider organization of which she is a part that any real notion of practitioner-centred non-participant observation is possible.

She might, for example, sit in as an observer on meetings that she is not usually party to, or she might observe the behaviour of nurses in situations in which she is not directly involved. However, this study of people and events which have no immediate bearing on the practitioner–researcher herself is not the main focus of PCR, and direct observation of this kind is therefore rare.

There are times, however, when some form of quantitative data about the behaviour of the practitioner–researcher would be useful. For example, she might be interested in the number of times that she touches her patient during a counselling session, or the duration of eye contact whilst carrying out a clinical procedure, and the only feasible way of collecting such data is by direct third party observation.

The use of third parties as data collectors goes somewhat against the spirit of PCR, but the usefulness of the data might well override any methodological objections. The most obvious and relevant person to draft in as non-participant observer would be a colleague, since she will be familiar with the clinical setting and will be least likely to misinterpret the situation she is observing.

Non-participant, direct observation is therefore one of the few times in PCR (along with the example of interviewing discussed earlier) when the data are collected by someone other than the practitioner–researcher herself. However, as we have seen, this objection is offset by the fact that direct observation is one of the few tools available to the case-study researcher which permits the collection of quantitative data.

As an example of the collection of quantitative data, Adams and Biddle (1970) carried out an educational study of 16 classrooms in which they attempted to measure the number and variety of 'incidents' or behaviours during 32 lessons. A structured tool was employed to collect two kinds of data: an incident count, which simply counted the number of separate occurrences; and a duration count, which registered the time span of each incident. As Cohen and Manion (1985) pointed out:

> Computer analysis later provided data on the number of incidents and the total amount of time spent on each kind of behaviour. Thus a complete record was accumulated of all instances of particular activities. ... showing the number of times that an activity occurred and how long it lasted.

It is easy to see how such an approach could be applied to clinical nursing settings, although such situations tend to be rather less structured than classrooms.

The strength of direct observation, however, is in its ability to obtain a numerical measure not only of quantity (that is, how *often* an event takes place), but also of quality (that is, how *effective* the event was). Unlike in the field of education, there are relatively few tools for formally assessing the quality of nursing situations, but one notable exception is dementia care mapping (DCM).

DCM (Kitwood and Bredin, 1994) employs time sampling and a structured coding frame for the study of the care provided to people with dementia in residential settings. Recordings are made at

5-minute intervals of the activity engaged in by the patient and of the perceived quality of that activity, and in this way a comprehensive map of the patient's day is built up, consisting of numerical and descriptive data which can later be shared with the ward team.

As with other forms of case-study research, there are a number of problems associated with non-participant observations. First, there is the objection that the researcher cannot possibly understand the situation she is observing, since she is standing outside it, or at least that there is 'the possibility ... of misunderstanding due to unfamiliarity with the culture and the language employed' (May, 1993). Burgess (1984) referred to this as ethnocentrism, pointing out the danger that 'the researcher may reject the informant's views without ever getting to know them'. However, this objection is minimized in PCR if a colleague who knows the practitioner well is employed to make the observations.

Secondly, as Hammersley and Atkinson (1983) pointed out, 'there may be severe limits on what can and cannot be observed and the questioning of participants may be impossible'. However, this is only a serious criticism if non-participant observation is the sole method of data collection, and as Nisbet and Watt pointed out, it is best seen as complementing other methods rather than competing with them.

Thirdly, the use of structured data collection tools such as DCM requires extensive training and can be extremely time consuming. However, little can be done to reduce this problem, and the quality of the data collected is a direct reflection of the care and time taken to collect it.

Participant observation

Although all of the above methods have a role to play, the most important method, indeed, the defining characteristic of reflective case-study research is participant observation. From this perspective, the reflective case study has more in common with ethnography than with traditional case-study methodology, with 'in the field' participant observation providing the main source of data and the other methods such as document analysis, interviews and non-participant observation being triangulated to provide support and validation for the study.

However, when the practitioner–researcher takes on the role of participant observer, she does so in a very peculiar way: as both clinician and researcher into her own clinical work, she is, in effect, a participant observer of her own practice. This role is rather different from the traditional role of participant observer, which has been defined as:

> the process in which an investigator establishes a many-sided and relatively long-term relationship with a human association in its natural setting, for the purposes of developing a scientific understanding of that association.
>
> (Lofland and Lofland, 1984)

Becker (1958) described how that 'scientific understanding' comes about:

> The participant observer gathers data by participating in the daily life of the group or organization he studies. He watches the people he is studying to see what situations they ordinarily meet and how they behave in them. He enters into conversation with some or all of the participants in these situations and discovers their interpretations of the events he has observed.

Hammersley and Atkinson (1983) challenged the above distinction between the researcher and the situation she is researching, claiming that the researcher is intrinsically and inescapably a part of the situation. Furthermore, they laid the foundations, albeit unintentionally, for the role of the practitioner–researcher as participant observer. Thus:

> We act in the social world and yet are able to reflect upon ourselves and our actions as objects in that world. By including our own role within the research focus and systematically exploiting our participation in the world under study as researchers, we can develop and test theory without futile appeals to empiricism, of either positivist or naturalist varieties.
>
> (Hammersley and Atkinson, 1983)

This is precisely what the practitioner–researcher hopes to achieve from participant observation: a reflection upon herself and her actions as a way of developing and testing theory. And reflection, of course, is the key to the whole process. When she is in the clinical setting, the practitioner–researcher is too busy practising also to observe her practice, and must rely on the reflective process, Schön's reflection-on-action, in order to extract the data from the situation at a later time. In this, she is no different from the traditional participant observer, who is too busy participating in the situation to record her observations at the time and has to sit down after the event in order to write up her fieldnotes.

However, as Van Manen (1990) pointed out, there is also a logical reason why the practitioner–researcher cannot reflect on her practice while it is taking place, since this would involve consciousness itself as the object of consciousness, which would in turn modify or change that which she was seeking to reflect on. Van Manen gave a simple example to illustrate his argument:

> A person cannot reflect on lived experience while living through the experience. For example, if one tries to reflect on one's anger while being angry, one finds that the anger has already changed or dissipated. Thus, phenomenological reflection is not *introspective* but *retrospective*. Reflection on lived experience is always recollective; it is reflection on experience that is already passed or lived through.

The basic tool of participant observation for the practitioner–researcher, and indeed of reflective case-study methodology as a whole, is therefore reflection-on-action, 'the retrospective contemplation of practice undertaken in order to uncover the knowledge used in a particular situation, by analyzing and interpreting the information recalled' (Fitzgerald, 1994). The problem, however, is that reflection-on-action as a form of practice development is a relatively informal process, whereas what is required for reflective case-study research is a formal data collection method.

Van Manen (1990) believed that he had discovered such a method in the act of writing, or what he referred to as 'textual labor'. Reflection, he argued, demands a certain form of consciousness, 'a consciousness that is created by the act of literacy: reading and writing'. Thus, 'writing is closely fused into the research activity and reflection itself'.

This view would appear to conflict with what we might term the 'Martini' approach to reflection, that it can be done 'anytime, any place, anywhere', an approach exemplified in the work of Chris James (Clarke *et al.*, 1994). However, as Andrews (1996) pointed out, 'reflection is ... not to be confused with thinking about practice, which may only involve recalling what has occurred rather than learning from it'. It is important, therefore, that we distinguish between the act of thinking about our practice and the act of learning from those thoughts.

In fact, both of these activities are relevant to the practitioner–researcher, and represent different stages of the research process. Thinking about practice is a natural psychological activity of free association which can indeed be done almost anywhere and at any time, and corresponds to the data collection stage of research. From the perspective of participant observation and reflective case-study methodology, it involves recalling the details of the features of practice relevant to our enquiry, thinking about how it could have been done differently, or about the aspects which were particularly successful.

Indeed, many psychologists would argue that it is not only a natural process, but one that is essential to our psychological well-being. We have probably all walked home after a bad day at work reflecting on an interaction that went particularly badly, thinking about what we should have said, and fantasizing a successful outcome. Similarly, we have all mentally replayed a successful nursing intervention, perhaps in response to a crisis, congratulating ourselves on a job well done.

However, this process of recollective reflection merely provides us with the raw data of our experiences. In order to use those experiences creatively, that is, to transform them into experiential knowledge, a further stage is required, and this is the stage of creative reflection which Bamberger and Schön (1991) described as 'conversing with [the] materials', and which Van Manen referred to as 'textual labor'. He continued:

> Writing fixes thought on paper. It externalises what in some sense is internal; it distances us from our immediate lived involvements with the things of our world. As we stare at the paper, and stare at what we have written, our objectified thinking stares back at us. Thus, writing creates the reflective cognitive stance that generally characterizes the theoretic attitude in the social sciences. The object of human science research is essentially a linguistic project: to make some aspect of our lived world, of our lived experience, reflectively understandable and intelligible.
>
> (Van Manen, 1990)

The act of writing is more than merely transferring the thoughts from our head onto paper: it is a creative act in which knowledge is constructed out of our recollected data, and 'not until we had written this down did we quite know what we knew' (Van Manen, 1990).

This creative process of knowledge construction bears a striking similarity to the early behaviourists' description of creativity and innovation:

> One natural question often raised is, how do we ever get new verbal creations such as a poem or a brilliant essay? The answer is that we get them by manipulating words, shifting them about until a new pattern is hit upon ... How do you suppose Patou builds a new gown? Has he any "picture in his mind" of what the gown is to look like when it is finished? He has not ... He calls his model in, picks up a new piece of silk, throws it around her, he pulls it in here, he pulls it out there ... He manipulates the material until it takes on the semblance of a dress ... Not until the new creation aroused admiration and commendation,

both his own and others, would manipulation be complete ... The painter plies his trade in the same way, nor can the poet boast of any other method.

(Watson, 1925)

Lest you write this off as mechanical and reductionist, here is C. Wright Mills, one of the most creative postwar sociologists, talking about what he called 'intellectual craftsmanship':

> As you rearrange [your writings], you often find that you are, as it were, loosening your imagination. Apparently this occurs by means of your attempt to combine various ideas and notes on different topics. It is a sort of logic of combination, and "chance" sometimes plays a curiously large part in it.
>
> (Mills, 1959)

It is clear that these two very disparate writers, a behavioural psychologist and an anti-empirical sociologist, are saying much the same thing: that creative ideas occur at the time of the mechanical process of giving them shape. Our prior reflections are the raw materials, but they are only turned into knowledge as we write.

And we do not usually get it right the first time. Watson's dress designer manipulates the silk until he comes up with something original; Mills' intellectual craftsman (*sic*) rearranges her writing and combines various ideas until a new focus emerges, often largely by 'chance'. It is not chance, of course, or else we would all be famous dress designers and sociologists. But the point is that ideas often only crystallize during the physical act of writing them down.

Writing is therefore the method by which the practitioner–researcher turns the reflective data from participant observation of her own practice into experiential knowledge. Further advice on how to go about this creative process is difficult to give, since in the terminology of this book, it is experiential practical knowledge which each individual must discover for herself by *doing*. All I can do is to suggest the last three of the 'six golden rules for writing' offered by Ernest Gaines: 'Read read read, write write write'. In fact the importance of writing and rewriting cannot be overstated, and as Becker (1986) noted:

> you have already made many choices when you sit down to write, but probably don't know what they were. That leads, naturally, to some confusion, to a mixed-up early draft. But a mixed-up early draft is no cause for shame. Rather, it shows you what your early choices were, what ideas, theoretical viewpoints, and conclusions you had already committed yourself to before you began writing. Knowing that you will write many more drafts, you know that you need not worry about this

one's crudeness and lack of coherence. This one is for *discovery*, not *presentation*.

At the data collection stage, every draft is for discovery, and the more we write, the more we discover. The need for a large number of drafts also highlights the importance of a word processor as an essential data analysis tool, and one wonders how writers such as C. Wright Mills and Howard Becker ever managed without one.

This process of recollective reflection followed by creative reflection can therefore be seen as the practitioner–researcher's method of participant observation, the equivalent in traditional ethnography of writing up fieldnotes. Clearly, it is a very intense and time-consuming activity, and there are other less demanding ways in which the data from recollective reflection can be transformed into knowledge. One of these is through clinical supervision, which has been described as:

> a meeting between two or more people who have a declared interest in examining a piece of work. The work is presented and they will together think about what was happening and why, and what was done or said, and how it was handled, could it have been handled better or differently, and if so how?
>
> (Wright, 1992)

Clinical supervision might, from the above description, be seen as the reflective equivalent of the semi-structured or unstructured interview, in which data about the practice situation are obtained through a verbal exchange or 'conversation with a purpose'. It is therefore closely linked with the method of asking a colleague to interview you which we discussed earlier.

Similarly, critical incident analysis, the use of structured guidelines for the recording of clinical incidents, might be thought of as a form of retrospective structured non-participant observation in which the practitioner–researcher is herself the retrospective observer of her own practice rather than a colleague or other external person. However, although these methods require far less effort than 'textual labor', the rewards are correspondingly less enlightening. In research, as in most creative activities, what you get out is a direct function of the amount of time and effort that you put in. Now look at the Reflective Break on page 156.

Reflective participant observation of your own practice is the most important, valuable and rewarding data collection method available in reflective case-study research, and has a number of advantages over traditional forms of participant observation. Sapsford and Abbott (1992) summarized these as:

REFLECTIVE BREAK

REFLECTIVE WRITING

Write a reflective account of a specific incident based on a participant observation of your own practice. Try to be as critical and analytical as possible.

Now reflect on the act of writing the account. To what extent did you plan what you were going to write beforehand? Did anything emerge while you were writing that you had not planned to write? Were you surprised by the outcome?

The major advantage is that you already have a natural role, the one you are carrying out in your job. There is no question of "joining" or "passing": you are already *in*. Equally important, at a practical level, you have no need to find your way through a maze of "gatekeepers": you are already in the situation and can take whatever notes it pleases you to take with no need for anyone's permission.

But as well as being the most rewarding method in reflective case-study research, it is also potentially the most dangerous. As Sapsford and Abbott went on to warn:

> It can be destructive of relationships, it can upset and sidetrack your professional practice, and the "methodological imagination" can sometimes be stretched to the point where your very sense of identity comes under attack.

They continued by identifying a number of difficulties that the practitioner–researcher is likely to encounter, including:

- the difficulty in "standing back" from the situation in which the practice/research is taking place;
- the difficulty in putting aside your own values and goals for the duration of the study;
- the difficulty in being perceived by colleagues as probing or prying into their practice and their relationships;
- the difficulty in questioning your own beliefs and the possibility of "losing faith" in your own practice.

(Sapsford and Abbott, 1992)

There are no easy solutions to these problems, but there are two things which the practitioner–researcher can do which might help to minimize them. First, she should negotiate with her colleagues *before* the study commences. Despite the earlier comment by Sapsford and Abbott that she can take whatever notes she pleases, it is good manners as well as good practice to seek permission from colleagues and managers just like in any other participant observation study. It is also wise to establish some ground rules, particularly with respect to confidentiality.

Secondly, as Sapsford and Abbott remind us, research supervision is probably more necessary with reflective participant observation than with any other method of data collection. Thus:

> It is not a form of research to be undertaken without supervision from someone who has been 'in the field' and knows the problems, and from an academic base where, at frequent intervals, you can change roles and discharge the tensions and self-doubts which have accumulated during the fieldwork. (Sapsford and Abbott, 1992)

This issue of supervision and where to get it will be discussed later in the chapter.

Validity and reliability

The previous chapter showed that the issues of internal validity (the degree to which we are measuring what we claim to be measuring) and reliability (the accuracy of those measures and their consistency over time) of single-case experimental research were fairly straightforward. However, with reflective case-study research the issues are rather more complex.

The scientific view of validity and reliability

Yin (1994) attempted to apply the traditional scientific validity criteria to case studies, pointing out that they are often criticized for failing to develop a sufficiently operational set of measures and for employing subjective judgements in the collection of data. The problem is that whereas in traditional scientific research, some degree of validity is guaranteed by the use of previously validated instruments, the data collection methods of case-study research are not readily subject to such tests.

For example, the usual way of validating a new attitude scale would be to administer the new test, along with an already valid existing test, to a group of subjects and to statistically correlate the two sets of data. If there is a close correlation between the scores on the two tests, then we could say with some confidence that the new scale is measuring the same construct as the already validated one. If there is little correlation, then either the new test is measuring something different, or else it is not measuring anything at all.

Clearly, however, interviews and participant observations are not open to the same validity checks, and an alternative must be found. Yin suggested that the internal validity of case-study research could be maximized by triangulation, that is, the use of multiple sources of evidence, and also by allowing the informants to review a draft of the study before it is published. In this way, he claimed, any obvious anomalies will be detected and can be revised or reformulated.

Yin also considered the question of reliability, the objective of which he described as:

if a later investigator followed exactly the same procedures as described by an earlier investigator and conducted the same case study all over again, the later investigator should arrive at the same findings and conclusions.

(Yin, 1994)

Reliability, he concluded, could be ensured by making as many steps in the research process as operational as possible 'and to conduct research as if someone were always looking over your shoulder'. The aim is to write up the study in such a way that it could be easily repeated by another researcher, and:

a good guideline for doing case studies is therefore to conduct the research so that an auditor could repeat the procedures and arrive at the same results.

(Yin, 1994)

The problem, however, and one which Yin did not address, is that this strategy merely ensures that the issue of reliability *could* be addressed by repeating the study; it does nothing to ensure that the study *is*, in fact, reliable, and it is highly unlikely that anyone would actually bother to replicate a case study in this way.

Alternative approaches to validity and reliability

Whereas Yin was concerned with the scientific credibility of case-study research, other writers have argued that traditional scientific concepts of validity and reliability simply do not apply.

What estimates of reliability can be given for a field-note jotted down in the chaos of a classroom discussion? What is the validity of an interpretation which comes like a blinding flash on the train home from a field visit?

(Kemmis, 1980)

Thus, in contrast to Yin's claim that reliability could be ensured by providing enough information for a study to be repeated, Hamilton (1980) argued that the whole notion of replication in case-study research is meaningless.

It is possible to state that two studies produced identical results. It is never possible to say they were conducted under identical conditions: if they were conducted at the same time, they must have occupied different places; if they were conducted at the same place they must have occurred at different times.

Each case study is unique and cannot be repeated, and the whole issue of reliability in case-study research is therefore redundant.

We will turn now to the issue of validity, and in particular to internal construct validity, which Hammersley and Atkinson (1983) saw in terms of whether the data generated by the study could be said to support the theoretical concepts being postulated by the researcher; that is, could the researcher be justified in constructing *this* theory from *these* data? They pointed out that the issue is not as straightforward as in traditional scientific research, where either data are generated first and then used to construct a theory (induction), or else a theory is postulated and data are then obtained to test it (deduction).

In case study, however, data and theory are developed reflexively at the same time, and 'there is an interplay between finding indicators [data] and conceptualizing the analytic categories [theories]' (Hammersley and Atkinson, 1983). It makes no sense, therefore, to talk of the study measuring the constructs it was designed to measure, since those constructs are not known at the outset, and only become apparent as the study progresses. Thus, the theoretical constructs of the study are as much *determined* by the emerging data as they are *supported* by them, and:

> it is only when the analysis is written up that the relationship between concept and indicator becomes an asymmetrical one, with the latter serving as evidence that the claims made by means of the concept are valid.
>
> (Hammersley and Atkinson, 1983)

Hammersley and Atkinson were critical of Yin's concept of respondent validation, claiming that:

> we cannot assume that any actor is a privileged commentator on his or her own actions, in the sense that an account of the intentions, motives, or beliefs involved are accompanied by a guarantee of their truth.
>
> (Hammersley and Atkinson, 1983)

The respondent's account is neither more valid than the researchers, nor is it necessarily more truthful, since 'it may be in a person's interests to misinterpret or misdescribe his or her own actions, or to counter the interpretations of the ethnographer'. Thus:

> Whether respondents are enthusiastic, indifferent or hostile, their reactions cannot be taken as direct validation or refutation of the observer's inferences. Rather, such processes of so-called "validation" should be treated as yet another valuable source of data and insight.
>
> (Hammersley and Atkinson, 1983)

They did, however, support Yin's use of triangulation as a test of validity, but developed it further to include:

- Data source triangulation, the comparison of data from different phases of the fieldwork or different participants.
- Triangulating between researchers, which is not particularly relevant to reflective case-study research as it is usually conducted only by the practitioner–researcher.
- Technique triangulation, the comparison of data derived from different research methods.

We can see, then, that Yin's respondent validation is not in itself a method of validation, but merely provides one source of data for data source triangulation.

A more radical view than that outlined above suggests that the validity of case-study research is ascribed by the reader. Adelman *et al.* (1976) claimed that case studies offer a 'surrogate experience' in which validity is attained by 'the shock of recognition'. It is the reader's responsibility to decide whether the case is a valid one, and the researcher therefore has a responsibility to present a rounded and comprehensive report in which conflicting viewpoints, including the viewpoint of the researcher herself, are represented in a balanced way.

Kemmis (1980) preferred the term 'authority' to validity, and claimed that the authority of a case report depends on it being 'authentic' and 'reasonable'. Only if it is an authentic account, grounded in the circumstances of the reader's life, will it be comprehensible, and only if it presents 'good reasons' for the particular structure and course of action of the study will it be acceptable to the reader.

In fact, Kemmis argued that authority goes beyond validity. A valid study is one in which there is a congruence between data and theory, where the researcher is justified in drawing the conclusions she does from the findings she has generated. An authoritative study, on the other hand, communicates more than it says by appealing to the tacit knowledge of the reader through what Kemmis called 'rich description'. Thus:

> Rich description of action-contexts creates the conditions for imagining what cannot be stated propositionally: it allows the reader to imagine himself in the social world of the case studied.
>
> (Kemmis, 1980)

Validity is transcended, the link between data and theory is broken, and the reader is invited to construct her own theoretical account of the case.

Maximizing validity

Having discussed a number of different concepts of validity in case-study research, I will end this section with some considerations for maximizing the validity of a study. Bruyn (1966) outlined six indices of 'subjective adequacy' which he believed would enhance the validity of observational research.

1 *Time:* the more time that an observer spends with a group, the greater the "subjective adequacy" or validity of the study.
2 *Place:* validity is enhanced by a familiarity with the physical environment in which the study takes place.
3 *Circumstances:* The more varied the observer's opportunities to relate to the group, both in terms of status, role and activities, the greater will be her understanding.
4 *Language:* The more familiar that the researcher is with the language of the social setting, the more accurate will be her interpretation of that setting. This applies not only to verbal communication, but to non-verbals such as facial expressions and bodily gestures.
5 *Intimacy:* The greater the personal involvement with the group and its members, the more the researcher is able to understand the meanings and actions they undertake.
6 *Social consensus:* The greater the ability to understand the rules of a social setting, the easier it will be to communicate them to others.

(Bruyn, 1966)

In traditional case-study research, these six indices of subjective adequacy develop over time. However, when the practitioner–researcher is exploring her own practice in her own clinical setting, all six indices are enhanced by her favoured position within the organization. Whatever the problems of PCR, then, its validity is maximized because the researcher is already familiar with, and accepted in, the research setting.

Data analysis

Data analysis is the most difficult and obscure aspect of case-study research. Yin described analysis of case study material as 'examining, categorizing, tabulating, or otherwise recombining the evidence to address the initial propositions of a study' and went on to offer two strategies for focusing on the analysis.

First, as the above description suggests, we can employ the theoretical propositions which led to the case study in the first place, and which are represented by the objectives of the study and the research questions. For example, a case study to explore why the practitioner–researcher becomes angry with patients who have attempted suicide would focus the analysis on possible reasons for her anger and her patients' reactions to it.

Secondly, where such theoretical propositions have not been made explicit at the outset of the study, we can develop a descriptive framework which covers a range of topics relevant to the focus of the study. In a case study of why people attempt suicide, these might include analyses of suicide attempts in people who are depressed; of suicide attempts in people who are suffering from schizophrenia; of suicide attempts in people who are suffering from manic depressive psychosis, and so on.

However, these strategies only provide a framework for the analysis, and give little help with the process itself, which as Yin pointed out, has not been well defined in the past. Nisbet and Watt (1979), for example, spoke only of a deep level of theoretical analysis in which generalizations must be supported by evidence, but gave no indication as to how such an analysis might be conducted. Hammersley and Atkinson (1983), however, maintained that data analysis should not be treated as 'a mysterious process about which little can be said and no guidance given', and outlined a number stages of analysis beyond the level of simple description, culminating in the development of a theory or theories.

First, the researcher must familiarize herself with the data through a careful reading of it, and 'at this stage the aim is to use the data to think with' (Hammersley and Atkinson, 1983). They continued:

> One looks to see whether any interesting patterns can be identified; whether anything stands out as surprising or puzzling; how the data relate to what one might have expected on the basis of common-sense knowledge, official accounts, or previous theory; and whether there are any apparent inconsistencies or contradictions among the views of different groups or individuals, or between people's expressed beliefs or attitudes and what they do.

This stage begins early in the research process and contributes to the ongoing planning and implementation of the study, unlike traditional scientific research, where data analysis usually takes place only after all the data have been collected. The outcome of this stage is a number of what Blumer (1954) called 'sensitizing concepts' which give the researcher 'a general sense of reference and guidelines' and provide the focus for further data collection and analysis.

The second stage is to begin to develop the analytical categories which emerge from these sensitizing concepts into a theoretical scheme, 'finding links between the concepts and adding new ones' (Hammersley and Atkinson, 1983). One approach to this is to employ what Glaser and Strauss (1967) called the 'constant comparative method' in which each segment of data is compared with all the other segments in the same category or categories. As Hammersley and Atkinson noted, 'as this process of systematic sifting and comparison develops, so the emerging model will be clarified'. They further pointed out that this method is not purely inductive, and that the researcher brings her own knowledge and bias to the process of theory building, and should approach the data with a number of different perspectives and hypotheses in mind.

Once the researcher has constructed a number of analytical categories, the next stage is the development of typologies in which 'a set of phenomena is identified that represents subtypes of some more general category' (Hammersley and Atkinson, 1983). Lofland (1970) suggested that typologies are developed in four stages:

1 by "self-consciously" assembling all the relevant data at the researcher's disposal;
2 by teasing out variations in those data;
3 by classifying the variations into an articulate set of types;
4 by presenting the types to the reader "in some ordered and preferably named and numbered manner".

Hammersley and Atkinson pointed out the danger of generalizing typologies beyond the limits of the available data, and stressed the importance of constantly referring back to that data, and this is the point at which the concerns of analysis and validation merge: validation takes place during the process of analysis, and analysis is part and parcel of validation.

Often, the development of typologies, in which the data are ordered, named and numbered, will represent the end-point of the case study, but there might be occasions where the aim is theory construction. In fact, as Hammersley and Atkinson pointed out, the issue is not so much one of theory *construction*, which is a relatively simple step on from a typology, but of theory *testing*, and they suggested Denzin's method of 'analytic induction' as best suited to the purpose. Denzin (1978) outlined the stages of analytic induction as follows:

1 A rough definition of the phenomenon to be explained is formulated.
2 An hypothetical explanation of that phenomenon is formulated.
3 One case is studied in the light of the hypothesis with the object of determining whether the hypothesis fits the facts in that case.
4 If the hypothesis does not fit the facts, either the hypothesis is reformulated or the phenomenon to be explained is redefined, so that the case is excluded.
5 Practical certainty may be attained after a small number of cases has been examined, but the discovery of negative cases disproves the explanation and requires a reformulation.
6 This procedure of examining cases, redefining the phenomenon, and reformulating the hypothesis is continued until a universal relationship is established, each negative case calling for a redefinition or a reformulation.

If this process of theory construction looks familiar, it is because it has already been explored earlier in the book, where it was referred to as analytical generalizability.

Data analysis in case-study research is a difficult and complex process, and although it might help to follow a strategy such as that outlined above, a great deal of the skill involved derives from tacit knowledge that can be learned but cannot be taught. Yin (1994) maintained that 'much depends on an investigator's own style of rigorous thinking', whereas Hammersley and Atkinson argued that data analysis is inextricably linked with the activity of writing. Thus:

> It is not altogether fanciful to suggest that the act of "interpretation" in interpretative sociology is as much an act of writing, of the organization of sociological texts, as it is a matter of cognitive processes of understanding.
>
> (Hammersley and Atkinson, 1983)

Barthes (1977) went even further, and argued that the processes of research and of writing are inseparable, and that 'research is then the name which prudently, under the constraint of certain social conditions, we give to the activity of writing'. This process of writing as knowledge generation has already been discussed in the section on participant observation, but at this stage in the case study it takes on a new significance. Thus:

> In writing, I tap my tacit knowledge. I externalize my thought-at-competence through my action-at-performance. My writing becomes both symbolic expression of thought (this is what I mean) and the critical reflection on that thought (do I really mean this?). My writing is

both reflection on action (what I have written) and reflection in action (what I am writing). The very act of making external, through the process of writing, what is internal, in the process of thinking, allows me to formulate explicit theories about the practices I engage in intuitively.

(McNiff, 1990)

For the practitioner–researcher who is carrying out a study into her own practice for her own benefit, the notion that the analysis continues into the writing-up stage provides the main justification for writing-up the study at all. She is, after all, writing primarily for herself, and if writing-up was merely an exercise in data recording, the field notes would suffice and there would be little point in producing a formal report. However, if we accept that writing is a process of creating knowledge as much as of recording it, then it is likely that new analytical insights will continue to emerge almost until the last word has been written. Thus, as Schatzman and Strauss (1973) pointed out:

In preparing for any telling or writing, and in imagining the perspective of his specific audience, the researcher is apt to see his data in new ways: finding new analytic possibilities, or implications he has never before sensed. This process of late discovery is full of surprises, some- times even major ones, which lead to serious reflection on what one has "really" discovered. Thus, it is not simply a matter of the researcher writing down what is in his notes or head; writing or telling as activities exhibit their own properties which provide conditions for discovery.

It might be as well, then, to end this section with some advice on the structure of the written report,[4] and probably the most comprehensive and practical assistance is provided by Yin (1994), who offered six possible structures:

1 Linear-analytic structures in which the sequence of subtopics involves the issue or problem being studied, a review of the relevant prior literature, the methods used, the findings from the data collected and analyzed, and the conclusions and implications from the findings. Many readers will recognise this as the standard format for scientific reports.
2 Comparative structures in which the same case study is repeated two or more times, comparing alternative descriptions or explanations of the same case.
3 Chronological structures where the sequence of chapters might follow the early, middle and late phases of a case history.
4 Theory-building structures in which the sequence of chapters will follow some theory-building logic, with each chapter unravelling a new part of the theoretical argument.

5 Suspense structures, which invert the analytic approach by presenting the outcome of the study first and then developing an explanation of that outcome along with alternative explanations.
6 Unsequenced structures in which the sequence of chapters assumes no particular importance, and which are usually employed in descriptive studies.

You should not feel that you have to follow any of the above structures; many studies mix and match, or evolve their own structure to meet their own idiosyncratic needs. Also, beware of overly 'tidying up' the account by tying up loose ends that would be better off remaining loose.

There are also several stylistic points to consider when writing-up. May (1993) suggested writing in the first person, and this is particularly appropriate for the practitioner–researcher, who is not only writing about what she did as a researcher, but probably also about her own practice. Wolcott (1990) argued that for congruence, the past tense should be used throughout, and not just in the account of the method, and Geertz (1973) advised that the report should include plenty of 'thick description', that is, specific instances from the field-notes.

Finally, the importance of revising and rewriting cannot be overstated, and 'corrections, additions, revising and editing of the text are all part of the writing process through which everyone has to travel' (May, 1993).

Summary

Reflective case-study research borrows its methodology and methods from clinical psychology and anthropology. However, these disciplines are concerned with objectivity and with limiting the impact of the researcher on the setting she is studying. This, of course, is in stark contrast to the paradigm of PCR, which is aimed precisely at studying the impact and influence of the practitioner–researcher on her own clinical setting.

Reflective case-study research therefore goes well beyond the traditional bounds of anthropology and ethnography and allows the practitioner–researcher reflectively to explore her own practice by combining 'external' quasi-objective data from interviews, document analysis and third-party observations of her practice with 'internal' subjective data from her own reflections-on-action.

The most relevant use of reflective case-study research is to answer exploratory questions which seek to explain or explore relationships between variables by the collection and analysis of predominantly qualitative data. It can be employed to:

- describe a clinical situation;
- understand ourselves and our practice;
- formulate and test theories.

The predominant research strategy is the triangulation of a number of methods, what Yin referred to as 'converging lines of enquiry', within a single- or multiple-case design. Whereas single-case design can help the practitioner–researcher to understand and explore her own practice, multiple-case design allows her to develop, shape and refine theory. Reflective case study is therefore a powerful tool in the repertoire of the practitioner–researcher.

The data collection methods employed in reflective case-study research are often significantly modified from the traditional ethnographic approach. For example, as well as interviewing significant others, the practitioner–researcher will also interview herself; rather than observe others, she will ask others to observe her; and rather than participate in 'external' social and clinical situations in order to collect data, she will reflect on her own everyday participation in her own practice. This latter method of reflective participant observation is the most important and, indeed, the defining method of reflective case-study research.

This reflective and introspective approach to case-study research has a number of advantages and disadvantages over the more traditional methods, which have been explored in depth. It also requires a rather different approach to validating the findings, which is based on 'subjective adequacy' and a deep familiarity with the setting in which the research is taking place.

Notes for Chapter 5

1. Hammersley and Atkinson's book *Ethnography: principles in practice* is drawn on extensively in this chapter. It might seem odd to rely so heavily on a book about ethnography in a chapter about case-study methodology, especially given Yin's point about the confusion surrounding the two terms and my earlier distinction between PCR and ethnographic research. However, Hammersley and Atkinson rejected the naturalistic approach usually adopted by ethnographers for a reflexive view which recognized that:

all social research takes the form of participant observation: it involves participating in the social world, in whatever role, and reflecting on the products of that participation

(Hammersley and Atkinson, 1983)

Hammersley and Atkinson's reflexive ethnography is therefore closer to what this book has termed 'reflective case study research' than it is to traditional ethnography.

2. Marshall and Rossman (1989) pointed out that the complete list of sources of data is extensive, and includes films, photographs, video tapes, projective techniques, psychological testing, proxemics, kinesics, 'street ethnography' and life histories.

3. See MacDonald (1980) for an amusing exchange of letters between a case-study worker and the headmaster of the school where he is hoping to conduct his research, which nicely illustrates some of the pressures that can be brought to bear on the researcher.

4. Adelman *et al.* (1977) offered a variety of forms of reporting case-study research, including collage, film documentary, mixed-media presentations, role-play simulations, oral feedback and quasi-journalistic reports,as well as the more usual written reports. This account restricts itself to the latter.

REFLECTIVE BREAK

DESIGNING A REFLECTIVE CASE STUDY

Turn back to the environmental introspective exploratory questions that you formulated in the Reflective Break on page 93. Outline a reflective case study to answer that question under the following headings:

Problem to be addressed (e.g. what is the problem for *you* in *your* practice?)

Personal interest and prejudice in the problem

Research question (from the Reflective Break on page 93)

Research design (e.g. units of analysis, study propositions, single- or multiple cases)

Why is this design most appropriate for your research?

Data collection methods (e.g. documentation, archival records, interviews, observations, etc.)

Ethical and practical constraints

Expected outcomes

6

Reflexive action research

Background and rationale

Historical development

The history of action research is more a history of the different ways that the term has been used over the years than of the development of a single coherent methodology. As Winter (1987) pointed out in the introduction to his book:

> My argument can not begin by tracing a "history" nor by reviewing "the literature" of action-research, since that would be to presuppose a definition and a coherence for action-research whose absence, precisely, is the occasion for the work.

When we refer to action research, then, we are not referring to a single methodology, but to a 'terminological anarchism' (Kalleberg, 1990), and this makes it difficult to trace a precise history. However, it is important that we try, since the history of action research is the history of how an emerging, if diverse, group of methodologies has been developed in an attempt to meet the demands of the various disciplines which it serves. In order to determine an appropriate action research methodology for PCR, it is therefore necessary to examine these various strands and the ways that they meet (or do not meet) the requirements of their fields of practice. Thus, in contrast to Winter's view, 'in understanding the countenance of action research, one must understand the historical traditions of the movement and the diversity of approaches for doing action research' (McKernan, 1991).

Most writers agree that the founder of action research was Kurt Lewin, an American social psychologist, who used the term from about 1944 until his death in 1947. Lewin (1946) described action research as 'a way of generating knowledge about a social system while, at the same time, attempting to change it', and applied his new methodology to a variety of industrial problems including morale, absenteeism, productivity and industrial conflict.

Lewin's original conception of action research has been described as:

> a series of spiralling decisions, taken on the basis of repeated cycles of analysis, reconnaissance, problem reconceptualization, planning, implementation of social action, and evaluation regarding the effectiveness of action.
>
> (McKernan, 1991)

The philosophy underlying this action cycle was that a social process could be studied by introducing changes and scientifically observing the effects of those changes on the process. Furthermore, if the changes proved to be beneficial, the social situation being studied could be 'refrozen' in that improved state. Thus, for Lewin, action research fulfilled the dual purpose of social enquiry and social action, such that 'research that produces nothing but books will not suffice' (Lewin, 1948).

At the same time that Lewin was carrying out his studies in America, the Tavistock Institute of Human Relations in Britain was developing its own form of action research to address the problems of organizational consultancy, although as Hart and Bond (1995) pointed out, this strand of development was not acknowledged as action research until the 1960s. The Tavistock model was more openly confronting and therapeutic than Lewin's version of action research, and included 'a problem-centred approach, a commitment to establishing relationships with clients over time, a focus on client needs and an emphasis upon research as a social process' (Hart and Bond, 1995).

Following these innovations, action research was quickly adopted by the discipline of education, particularly in America (see, for example, Corey, 1953). Here, according to Sanford (1970), it flourished for 10 years before going into a decline brought about by a huge increase in funding for 'hard' scientific research. However, educational action research was revived in Britain in the early 1970s by the pioneering work of Lawrence Stenhouse and initiatives such as the Ford Teaching Project (Elliott, 1976–7). This revival, according to Edwards and Talbot (1994), came about

> in reaction to the increasing amount of research *on* teachers found in the late 1960s and 1970s and a tendency to turn these professionals into objects of study in ways that did little for the teaching profession.

We can see, then, that the philosophy underpinning action research in education was very different from either Lewin's industrial model which attempted to 'marry the experimental approach of social science with social action in response to major social problems of the day' (Kemmis, 1982), or the Tavistock model which was essentially consultative, and applied psychoanalytical theory to social problems.

In contrast, the emerging educational model sought to develop an alternative to the dominant scientific paradigm, and emphasized practitioner involvement and immediate local application. Stenhouse (1975) referred to this as the 'teacher as researcher' movement, characterized by collaborations between academic researchers and classroom-based practitioners.

However, Hart and Bond (1995) noted that by the late 1970s there was a growing dissatisfaction on the part of teachers with the 'expert' role of the outside academic researcher, and it was generally felt that the teachers' practice-based agendas were being neglected in favour of the generation and testing of scientific theory. This led Elliott (1978) to pioneer a reflective model of action research in which the roles of the researcher and practitioner finally merged and the goal of action research became professionalization. Thus:

> The major aim of action research is the establishment of conditions under which self-reflection is genuinely possible: conditions under which aims and claims can be tested, under which practice can be regarded strategically and 'experimentally', and under which practitioners can organize as a critical community committed to the improvement of their work and their understanding of it.
>
> (Kemmis, 1982)

This view of action research marked an important divergence from the traditional scientific research paradigm and fully established the role of the practitioner–researcher and the notion that theory could be generated *from* practice as well as being applied *to* it.

In nursing, action research only emerged as an accepted methodology in the mid 1980s (see, for example, Greenwood, 1984; Lathlean and Farnish, 1984). Sparrow and Robinson (1994) have argued that part of the reason for this late development has been nursing's obsession with emulating the research methodologies of the medical profession in an attempt to establish itself as an academic discipline, and it is only relatively recently that a widespread disillusionment with the positivist paradigm of medicine as being able to address problems of practice has begun to set in.

Action research approaches in nursing have therefore been developed first in an attempt to bridge the gap between theory and practice in a way that more traditional research methods seem unable to do (Webb, 1990), and secondly in recognition that the aims and practices – and hence the research methodologies – of nursing are different from those of medicine, that 'nursing is *a social practice* the central purpose of which is to bring about positive change in the health status of individuals and communities' (Greenwood, 1994, my emphasis). However, action research in nursing has yet to develop a distinctive focus, or even a rationale, in the way that educational action research has managed to do.

Definitions

It should not be surprising, in view of the variety of different strands of action research, that the task of achieving a consensus on its definition is almost impossible. The best that we can hope to achieve is a loose agreement on its defining characteristics, but even here we run into problems.

For example, there is a difference of opinion as to the primary aim of action research, with some writers arguing that the aim is to improve practice (notably Ebbutt, 1985; Elliott, 1991), some arguing that the aim is to increase knowledge and develop theory (Kemmis and McTaggart, 1982; Holter and Schwartz-Barcott, 1993, albeit for very different reasons) and yet others claiming that it should aim for both. We are therefore faced with such contradictory statements as:

> The fundamental aim of action research is to improve practice rather than to produce knowledge. The production and utilization of knowledge is subordinate to, and conditioned by, this fundamental aim.
>
> (Elliott, 1991)

and:

> The development of theory is the final goal of action research. The researcher develops new or expands or enhances already existing scientific theories.
>
> (Holter and Schwartz-Barcott, 1994)

There is similar disagreement as to the basic epistemological underpinnings of action research. Thus, Lewin (1948) saw action research as strongly scientific, as more recently did McKernan (1991); Cohen and Manion (1985) claimed that it 'interprets the scientific method much more loosely'; whilst Usher and Bryant (1989) and Winter (1987) saw it as rejecting the scientific paradigm entirely. Therefore, we are once again offered such contradictory assertions as:

> This by no means implies that the research needed [for action research] is in any respect less scientific or "lower" than what would be required for pure science in the field of social events. I am inclined to hold the opposite to be true.
>
> (Lewin, 1948)

and:

> action research is not located within a natural science paradigm and is not concerned to provide "scientific" explanations of the world or make a contribution to formal theory in foundation disciplines.
>
> (Usher and Bryant, 1989)

Even on the issue of collaboration, which almost all writers seem to agree is a feature of action research, closer examination reveals at least three different usages of the term. First, there are those like Lewin (1948) and Holter and Schwartz-Barcott (1993), who took it to mean collaboration between 'outside' academic researchers and 'inside' practitioners. Secondly, there are those like Reason (1988), who advocated for a collaboration between the researchers and the subjects of the research. Thirdly, there are those like Ebbutt (1985) and Carr and Kemmis (1986), who saw collaboration as between a number of individual practitioners involved in researching their own practice with no outside help from 'professional' researchers.

The one area of agreement would seem to be that action research operates in a succession of cycles or spirals which are initiated by a practical problem and include elements of understanding or theorizing, bringing about change by acting, and carrying out some form of formal or reflective research activity.

Even on this point, however, there is some dispute. For example, Cohen and Manion (1985) outlined an eight-point model which made no mention of an ongoing cyclical process, but rather described an 'eighth and final stage' which included 'the interpretation of the data; inferences to be drawn; and overall evaluation of the project'. But as Carr and Kemmis (1986) pointed out:

> In action research, a single loop of planning, acting, observing and reflecting is only a beginning; if the process stops there it should not be regarded as action research at all. Perhaps it could be termed "arrested action research".

There is clearly a serious lack of consensus on what action research is, on what are its aims and underlying principles, and on how it is to be conducted, and we have an opportunity, therefore, to tailor a methodology specifically to the needs of the practitioner–researcher. It will be recalled from Chapter 3 that what the reflexive practitioner requires from action research is a way of integrating practice and research in a single act whose aim is not primarily the generation of knowledge and theory but the implementation of clinical change, so that research becomes 'built-in' to practice and clinical change is built-in to research. This approach to research, where practice and research become two parts of the same act, will be referred to as reflexive action research.

Research questions

If the practitioner–researcher is concerned with research that is 'built in' to practice, then the impetus for research should be a problem that continues to resist resolution, or as Elliott (1991) put it, 'the feeling that some aspect(s) of a practice need to be changed if its aims and values are to be more fully realized'. The primary focus of reflexive action research is thus not research, but action, and the *form* which action research questions take is, in the terminology of this book, invariably developmental rather than descriptive or exploratory.

Developmental questions are 'how' questions (or as McNiff *et al.* put it, 'how can I improve?' questions) which are concerned with changing a situation, but that does not mean that the action researcher has no concern for theory. In reflexive action research, theory and action cannot be separated and theory either determines the nature of the initial action, or else theory emerges from the action. The point is, however, that the theory is merely instrumental and the main aim of reflexive action research is to bring about an improvement in practice.

Moving to the *focus* of the question, reflexive action research can ask either introspective questions which focus on the practitioner–researcher herself as a therapeutic agent; practice-based questions which focus on her clinical work or her relationships with her patients; or organizational questions which focus on care management issues.

And finally, the *subject* of reflexive action research can be either personal, relating to the practitioner–researcher's own practice, or

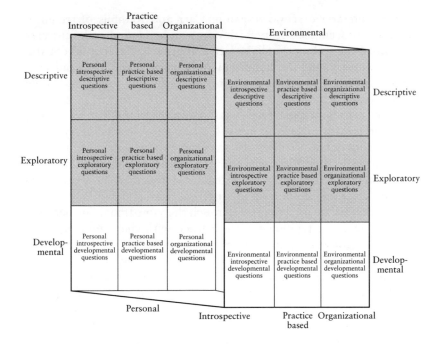

Figure 6.1   *Reflexive action research questions.*

environmental, relating to her working environment. The scope of reflexive action research questions is shown in Figure 6.1.

Methodology and research design

Typologies and methodologies of action research

As we have seen, there is no single methodology which satisfies all action researchers; indeed, there is not even a single component of a methodology on which there is unanimous agreement. This lack of consensus on even the basic tenets of action research has led a number of writers to formulate typologies which attempt to encompass the whole range of views and approaches under several broad headings.

Lewin, for example, distinguished between experimental, empirical, diagnostic and participative action research; McKernan wrote of scientific, practical-deliberative, critical-emancipatory and rational-interactive action research; Carr and Kemmis of technical, practical and emancipatory action research; Holter and Schwartz-Barcott of the technical collaborative approach, the mutual collaboration approach and the enhancement approach; and Hart and Bond of experimental, organizational, professionalizing and empowering action research.

Whereas each of these typologies is self-contained, has an internal logic and is fairly inclusive, each offers a more or less arbitrary way of categorizing what is, after all, a very broad range of disparate methodologies, and there is scope for enormous confusion and misunderstanding when they are considered together. In some cases, similar terms are employed in different ways, and in other cases different terms are used to refer to much the same thing. Furthermore, each of the above typologies is concerned with characterizing action research according to the underlying philosophy of the approach rather than according to how the research is carried out.

Before we become too embroiled in arguments about the merits and demerits of various typologies, however, it should be remembered that our concern here is to develop a *reflexive* action research methodology for the practitioner–researcher in the exploration of her own practice. In order to satisfy the needs of the practitioner–researcher as outlined in this book, reflexive action research should have the following characteristics:

- It is research carried out by practitioners into their own practice in response to a perceived problem.
- It brings about direct improvement in the situation being researched.
- It contributes (usually indirectly) to the personal knowledge and theory of the practitioner–researcher.
- It is a cyclical or spiral process in which the outcomes from one cycle inform and direct the next cycle.

It must be acknowledged that this conception of action research is rather different from most of those discussed earlier in this chapter. It discounts research in which an outside 'expert' is called in to assist the practitioner; research in which the aim is to test or generate 'scientific' generalizable knowledge and theory; and it even challenges the notion of action research as essentially collaborative, although we shall see later that it proposes a particular form of collaboration between individual practitioner–researchers, each engaged in their own projects.

From this perspective, none of the above typologies are appropriate, and whole categories (in particular, the 'scientific' or 'technical' ones) do not even qualify as reflexive action research. What is required, then, is a way of conceptualizing the various strands of, and approaches to, reflexive action research as it has been defined in this chapter, that is, as a problem-centred, cyclical research methodology in which the practitioner–researcher explores and implements new ways of resolving problematical issues for her own practice.

A systems approach to clinical problems

We have seen that for the practitioner–researcher, the impetus to carry out a piece of reflexive action research is being confronted with a problem which defies resolution. The first step in developing a reflexive action research methodology is therefore to understand how problems develop and how they might be resolved, and for this I will employ some ideas from systems theory and cybernetics, taken from the practice of family therapy.

Cybernetics, which is concerned with communication and information flow in complex systems, introduces the concept of the feedback loop as a way of explaining how problems develop. In simple terms, it suggests that when we take action to resolve a problem, that action is fed back to the problem situation in a simple reflexive loop (Figure 6.2a). The nature of the action therefore determines whether the problem is resolved, maintained or escalated.

If the action serves to reduce the problem, then we have a negative feedback loop (Figure 6.2b). Each time we travel round the loop with another response, the problem becomes smaller and smaller until it finally disappears. For example, if our problem is a leg ulcer, and our action is to apply wound care method X, then each application of X would result in the wound becoming smaller until it finally heals.

If, on the other hand, the action maintains the problem, then we have reached a state of homeostasis (Figure 6.2c). The action is not reducing the problem, but neither is it making it worse, and the problem will continue indefinitely. For example, the application of wound care method Y to the problem of the leg ulcer does not have a healing effect, and is just toxic enough to inhibit the natural healing powers of the body. The wound neither improves nor deteriorates, and the problem becomes chronic and protracted.

Finally, if the action worsens the problem, then we have a positive feedback loop (Figure 6.2d) in which each attempt at a solution serves to amplify the problem. For example, the application of wound care

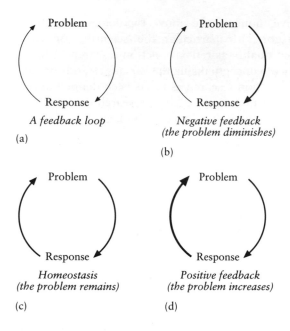

Figure 6.2   *A systems approach to clinical problems.*

method Z actually exacerbates the wound. The difficulty, however, is that often we do not recognize that the deterioration in the patient's condition is due to the treatment he is receiving, and we believe that he is getting worse *despite* the treatment rather than *because* of it. The response is then to increase the application of method Z, which makes the problem even worse, and so on in a vicious circle. In a positive feedback loop, therefore, the problem quickly escalates into a crisis. Now look at the Reflective Break on page 181.

Understanding-action-evaluation design

The aim of reflexive action research is to break into the feedback loop and modify the counter-productive 'solution' to the problem. There are a number of possible ways that this can be achieved, and thus a number of possible reflexive action research designs. The response of traditional action research is first an *understanding* of the problem in what Lewin described as a planning, theorizing and hypothesizing stage. This is followed by an *action* stage in which the theories are implemented or the hypotheses tested. Finally, there is an *evaluation*

REFLECTIVE BREAK

A POSITIVE FEEDBACK LOOP

Think of a situation from your own practice where things seemed to get worse despite your actions. Draw a simple systems diagram of the situation similar to the one shown in Figure 6.2d.

What could you do to improve the situation?

stage where the effects of the action are assessed, which in turn modifies the original problem. The cycle is then repeated until the problem is resolved. Thus, traditional action research:

> proceeds in a spiral of steps each of which is composed of a circle of planning, action, and fact-finding about the result of the action.
>
> (Lewin, 1946)

This traditional 'scientific' approach can also act as a model for reflexive action research, and will be referred to as the understanding-action-evaluation (UAE) design because of the sequence of the responses to the problem. It breaks into the positive feedback loop by first formulating a personal theory which attempts to understand why the action is not resolving the problem.

Once the reason for the maladaptive response is understood, it can then be altered in the action phase. It might only be necessary to stop doing it, that is, to do nothing, or else the maladaptive response might need to be replaced by a more appropriate one. Quite often, the most appropriate response is the exact opposite of the response which has unintentionally caused the problem, a so-called paradoxical intention (Frankl, 1973).[1]

Having taken action, its effect on the problem can then be evaluated, which in turn will modify the problem (hopefully for the better!). This process is shown in Figure 6.3, and is essentially the process of reflection-in-action or praxis which was outlined in Part One. Reflection-in-action can therefore be seen as a form of on-the-spot action research.

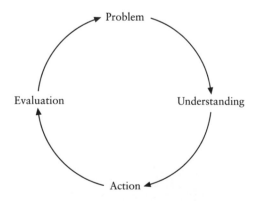

Figure 6.3   *UAE design.*

This research design will now be illustrated with an example from the practice of family therapy. The family in this example consisted of a husband and wife and their 15 year-old son. The parents identified the problem as the 'delinquent' behaviour of the boy, who was getting in with the wrong crowd and refusing to come home at his specified bed-time. The parents responded by getting tougher and tougher, and had now got to the point where they were locking the door and going to bed at midnight whether he was home or not. The action of a tough response was therefore maladaptive, and acting as positive feedback to the problem of 'delinquency', which was escalating out of control.

In order to resolve the problem, the situation was framed as a reflexive action research project with the personal practice-based developmental question: *how can I help this family to deal with their son's delinquent behaviour?*. From the perspective of the UAE action research design, the following plan was formulated:

Problem:
: The son was behaving in a way that was unacceptable to his parents. The more that the parents 'clamped down' on his behaviour, the worse it became.

Understanding:
: The personal theory was that the son was rebelling against parental authority. Therefore, the more that the parents tried to impose their authority, the more the son had to rebel against. The imposition of authority, which was seen by the parents as a solution to the problem, was in fact producing positive feedback and making the situation worse.

Action:
: The parents were told to stop trying to change their son's behaviour, in effect, to do nothing. This reduced the need, and indeed the opportunity, to rebel and diminished the problem behaviour. Alternatively, a 'paradoxical intention' could have been suggested, which would have involved asking the parents to do the opposite of what they were currently doing, in this case, to encourage the very behaviour which they were trying to reduce, which would have sanctioned the rebellion (thus, it would no longer *be* rebellion).

Evaluation: The parents were told to monitor their son's be-
                   haviour and to report back in 6 weeks, by which
                   time we would expect that the problem would have
                   resolved itself.

In this approach to action research, the action emerges from an
understanding of the problem, and is then evaluated according to
whether it resolves that problem. If the resolution is only partial, the
practitioner–researcher continues around the cycle until the problem
is eliminated or reduced to an acceptable level.

Action-evaluation-understanding design

Although the above UAE design forms the basis of traditional action
research, there are several other research designs which are appropriate for a reflexive problem-based approach. For example, there
will be occasions where an understanding of the problem is just not
possible, and in order to break the vicious circle on these occasions,
we might simply change our actions according to our intuition or
professional judgement. In other words, we do what feels to be the
right thing at the time and then attempt to understand our action by
evaluating its effects.

This model will be referred to as the action-evaluation-understanding (AEU) design (Figure 6.4) in which the vicious circle is
broken simply by doing something different and attempting to make
sense of it afterwards. As Dewey put it, 'we learn by doing and

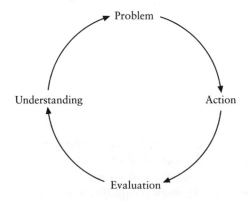

Figure 6.4   *AEU design.*

realizing what came of what we did'. For example, we might not understand how the response is positively reinforcing the behaviour, and it is only when we stop doing it or when we do the opposite and note its effect on the problem that we begin to understand its maladaptive effect.

Elliott (1991) described this approach to action research in the discipline of teaching:

> The teacher changes some aspect of his or her teaching in response to a practical problem and then self-monitors its effectiveness in resolving it. Through the evaluation the teacher's initial understanding of the problem is modified and changed. The decision to adopt a change strategy therefore precedes the development of understanding. Action initiates reflection.

Elliott added that this approach follows the natural logic of practical thinking, and that 'when practical problems arise, the practitioner's first priority is to act quickly in order to resolve it'. Thus, whereas UAE action research initially generates action out of theory, in the AEU design theory emerges from the action:

> The practice is the form of inquiry: a hypothetical probe into the unknown beyond one's present understanding, to be reviewed in retrospect as a means of extending that understanding. The search for understanding is carried out through changing the practice and not in advance of such changes.
>
> (Elliott, 1991)

This approach is the basis of reflection-on-action, in which an action, based on professional judgement, is taken in response to an immediate problem, and is later reflected on and learned from. For example, the practitioner–researcher does not understand why a patient is not responding to bereavement counselling, but her judgement tells her that he might prefer a less confronting approach. This problem could lead to her asking the personal practice-based developmental question: *how can I help this patient to open up more during counselling?* From this question, the following plan could be constructed:

Problem: Bereavement counselling is getting nowhere. The patient will not 'open up'.

Action: The practitioner–researcher takes a less confronting approach, giving the patient more psychological space.

Evaluation: The patient talks more and cries for the first time.

Understanding: The patient needed to feel less threatened in order to express his feelings.

In this case, the action was not based on a prior understanding of the problem. Rather, the understanding emerged from an evaluation of the modified action.

This design is also useful when the practitioner–researcher is addressing introspective questions, that is, questions about her own values, judgements and attitudes. Introspective developmental questions usually follow introspective exploratory questions; for example, the practitioner–researcher might first ask *why do I get angry at certain of my patients?* By carrying out a reflective case study, she might conclude that she gets angry because she is directing feelings of frustration about her own inabilities onto her patients. The introspective developmental question arising from this might therefore be *how can I stop projecting this anger I feel towards myself onto other people?*

Problem: I inappropriately become angry with some of my patients.

Action: When faced with these situations, I make a conscious effort to be less angry by, for example, telling myself that it is not the patient's fault.

Evaluation: I reflect on whether this has helped the situation.

Understanding: I now begin to understand how I might control my anger.

This situation is slightly different from the counselling example described previously because the practitioner–researcher enters this latter case with a good idea of what action needs to be taken. The research design therefore involves implementing the action and evaluating whether or not it is effective. If it is, then the reflective research from which the understanding arose is also validated in the process.

Evaluation-understanding-action design

A third reflexive action research design is necessary in situations

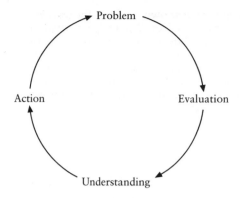

Figure 6.5   *EUA design.*

where neither action nor theory appears to be a viable first step, for example, in situations where the practitioner–researcher feels very unsure of what to do, or where an external gatekeeper to the research situation requests a more empirical approach. In cases such as these, we might initially respond with a formal, research-based evaluation of the problem, which in turn will lead to a theoretical understanding and to informed action. This will be referred to as the evaluation-understanding-action (EUA) design (Figure 6.5), in which the vicious circle is broken by a new intervention based on research. Elliott (1991) described this approach to action research in education:

> The teacher undertakes research into a practical problem and on this basis changes some aspect of his or her teaching. The development of understanding precedes the decision to change teaching strategies. In other words, reflection initiates action.

This design is more in keeping with the technical rationality paradigm, in which a research-based theory determines the action rather than being determined by it. Elliott (1991) pointed out that 'there is a theory of rational action here in which actions are selected or chosen on the basis of a detached and objective contemplation of the situation', and added that this design forms the basis on which Stenhouse originally conceptualized the notion of the 'teacher as researcher'.

Carr and Kemmis (1986) described a number of action research projects in education which followed this approach. For example:

Through close analysis of transcripts of their own teaching, the teachers involved discovered how their normal practices ... actually operated to deny students the opportunity to raise their own questions and to develop independence of their teacher in their learning.... The teachers learned to change the form of their classroom questioning, and to provide resources which encouraged students to raise questions in a framework of classroom activity which would give them opportunities to answer the questions they had raised.

(Carr and Kemmis, 1986)

To take a nursing example, a practitioner–researcher wishes to change the way that patients are admitted to her ward. She approaches the ward manager, who agrees that the current system is not working very well, but insists that any changes must be as a result of empirical research. The practitioner–researcher therefore formulates the environmental organizational developmental question *how can I improve the admission procedure on my ward?* and constructs the following plan:

Problem: The staff and patients seem dissatisfied with the current admission procedure.

Evaluation: Questionnaires and/or interviews are administered to evaluate the cause of the dissatisfaction.

Understanding: It emerges that currently the admission procedure takes place too soon after admission, and that patients would welcome the opportunity to settle in before being formally admitted.

Action: The admission procedure is modified to take account of the research findings.

As with all of the designs, however, this is not the end of the matter. The action will inevitably throw up some unforseen difficulties or will only partially resolve the problem, and several cycles are usually required before the problem is completely dealt with.

Summary

Three research designs have been outlined in response to the particular character and requirements of reflexive action research: the understanding-action-evaluation (UAE) design, the action-evaluation-understanding (AEU) design, and the evaluation-understanding-action (EUA) design, each of which offers a way of breaking the vicious circle or positive feedback loop of a clinical problem and a 'solution' which is actually maintaining the problem or making it worse.

Furthermore, each of these approaches is best suited to answering questions with a specific focus. The UAE design corresponds closest to the traditional practice development approach described by Lewin, and the most appropriate questions to be addressed by UAE action research are therefore what have been referred to as practice-based questions (see Figure 6.1). The AEU design, whilst able to address practice-based questions, is also suitable for introspective questions which focus on the internal world of the practitioner–researcher herself, on her beliefs, attitudes, skills, knowledge and expertise. Finally, the EUA design is best suited to answering organizational questions which require a more traditionally empirical focus.

Data collection methods

As we might expect from the 'methodological anarchism' described earlier, there is little consensus when it comes to data collection methods in action research. Some writers, for example, see action research as a particular kind of case study and advocate a rigorous programme of interviews, observations and questionnaires to uncover more or less objective knowledge (McKernan, 1991). Webb (1989) supported this view, arguing that action research should be eclectic but rigorous, and employ the methods most suitable for the subject under study.

At the other extreme, Edwards and Talbot (1994) have pointed out that:

> While accepting that some of the data will be objective in, for example, counts of the number of times a resource is used or in the content analysis of written text, we need to recognise that seeking objectivity is less of an issue for action researchers than for other researchers.

They suggested a wide range of methods including surveys, observation, interviews, life histories and repertory grids, and urged the researcher to adapt them creatively to her own particular needs, a view supported by Kalleberg (1990) who pointed out that 'in action research, we have the chance to try out new models, models that can often not be worked out in detail beforehand'. However, Edwards and Talbot focused on reflective diaries as the most important and relevant way of collecting data for action research projects, backed up with direct and unstructured observation. According to this view, then, action research is primarily a subjective process of exploring one's own practice.

Holter and Schwartz-Barcott (1993) adopted a compromise position, arguing that action research requires no particular model of data collection, while Hart and Bond (1995) added that:

> Action research may involve sophisticated types of quantitative evaluation designed to infer the relationship between cause and effect, or may use qualitative and/or much more informal means of evaluating processes, such as asking the participants directly for their comments on progress so far.

From the perspective of reflexive action research and the three designs described earlier, it is clear that we require a very eclectic approach to data collection similar to that advocated above by Hart and Bond. For example, if we wish to answer an introspective question using the AEU research design, we might employ a reflective diary as our main data collection instrument. If, on the other hand, we wish to answer an organizational question using the EUA design, we are more likely to employ a formal data collection method such as a questionnaire or interview.

McNiff *et al.* (1996) offered a very comprehensive summary of data collection methods for the reflexive action researcher who is concerned with exploring and improving her own practice, claiming that data can be collected by:

● Observing the effects of our actions on others and asking them to observe us.
● Asking other people for their views, and asking them for help in seeing their point of view.
● Looking for 'fingerprints' or evidence of our actions, which might include audio and video tapes, photographs or documents.

They went on to list a number of useful sources of data, including reflective journals, letters (to self and others), written reports to yourself, audio/videotaped conversations, comments by others on your performance, video recordings of current practice, questionnaires and fieldnotes.

Whereas access to some of these sources of data will entail the use of accepted and well tested social research methods, others will require a far more informal and *ad hoc* approach. It might seem strange to conduct a piece of research in which no formal data collection has taken place, and some readers will no doubt object that, in many cases, reflexive action research is not research at all, but merely a planned nursing intervention.[2]

However, it will be recalled that the aim of reflexive action research is for the practitioner–researcher to resolve a problem for her own practice by changing her response to that problem, thus breaking a vicious circle or positive feedback loop. The primary aim of reflexive action research is not to understand a problem, but to resolve it, and as Lewin (1948) pointed out, 'research that produces nothing but books will not suffice'. Reflexive action research is therefore defined and assessed not by the research methods employed, but by whether practice is systematically improved in a cycle of action, evaluation and understanding (but not, as we have seen, necessarily in that order). Reflexive action research is *action* research rather than action *research*.

Despite its action orientation, reflexive action research *could* involve the formal collection of empirical data. The practitioner-researcher might, for example, wish to explore how her practice could lead to a reduction in anxiety levels in patients about to undergo surgery, and she could evaluate whether an improvement has occurred by using a quantitative anxiety scale. The point, however, is that the formal collection and analysis of data is not an essential part of reflexive action research, and the data have no purpose other than to bring about improvements in the practice of the practitioner-researcher.

Validity and reliability

The aims of action research also have an important bearing on the way that its validity and reliability are assessed. For example, Usher and Bryant (1989) saw the purpose of action research as the generation of 'insider knowledge' which, they pointed out, makes it difficult to validate its truth claim to outsiders. Indeed, they went further to question whether action research can, or indeed should, attempt to justify itself to outsiders at all.

For Elliott (1991), who saw the primary aim of action research as improved practice, the validity of the theories it produces depended entirely on their 'usefulness in helping people to act more intelligently and skilfully'. Thus 'in action research "theories" are not validated independently and then applied to practice. They are validated through practice.' If the application of a theory leads to better practice, then the research which produced that theory, and the theory itself, can be said to be valid.

Greenwood (1994) made a similar point that action theories are simply 'chunks of practical reasoning', and that

> The propositions operational in practical reasoning are valid or true if they lead to the successful bringing about of the state of affairs that is desired.

However, this approach to validity maintains the gap between theory and practice in action research, and suggests that the theory can exist independently of the action to which it relates. Furthermore, it supports the technical rationality paradigm by implying that theories are applied to, and validated by, practice rather than being generated from them.

In reflexive action research, theory and action are intertwined, and must be validated together. Furthermore, the primary aim of the reflexive action researcher is to bring about improvements in her practice. Thus, whereas Elliott and Greenwood both saw the issue of validation as justifying the usefulness of a *theory* by applying it to practice, the primary concern of the reflexive action researcher is to validate the *action* component of the action research, that is, directly to validate the improvements to her practice. Seen from this perspective, the related issue of reliability, of the extent to which the data collection instruments measure consistently over time, is irrelevant since we are concerned with unique, one-off action projects rather than with the construction of enduring theory.

McNiff *et al.* (1996) probably best expressed the reflexive action research approach to validity when they wrote that 'validation enables action researchers to test their claims to have improved and understood better their own professional practice'. The research is valid if the researcher's claim to have improved her practice and to understand how and why those improvements came about is upheld by other people. Thus, 'making research public is the best way of getting it validated' (McNiff *et al.*, 1996), and this does not necessarily mean publishing it in a journal, but rather 'sharing the findings with other people, particularly colleagues in the work context, and checking with them whether your perceptions are reasonably fair and accurate'.

In fact, McNiff *et al.* suggested a number of different forums in which this validation could take place, and their suggestions are reproduced below in full:

Self-validation
As a responsible practitioner can you show to your own satisfaction that you have done the things you set out to do? Can you show that you have carried out a systematic enquiry, to help you live out your values more effectively than before? Can you offer a rational account of your own professional learning?

Peer validation
Can you convince a group of peers that your claim to knowledge is to be taken seriously? Will they agree that you are demonstrating responsible and excellent practice? Can you offer clear criteria for the assessment of your work, and produce unambiguous evidence around those criteria?

Up-liner validation
Can you show to managers and those in authority that you have intervened in your practice to improve it, and that your way of working could be adopted in institutional development plans?

Client validation
Will the people you are supporting agree that you have acted in their interests, and that the quality of their life is better because of your intervention?

Academic validation
This is validation by the academic community in terms of whether it agrees that you have contributed to a recognized body of knowledge. Many of you who are engaged in courses that lead to awards will have to submit your work for the established forms of examination.

The general public
Your final validation group will be the wider community of readers, in organizational or general contexts.

(McNiff *et al.*, 1996)

However, validation should not be left until the end of the project, and McNiff *et al.* (1996) suggested the formation of a validation group which 'could be made up of members from any of the groups listed above and may vary in size and formality'. The group should act as a 'sympathetic critic', and its role is to make recommendations to the researcher at each stage of the project in order to ensure that the research remains focused and on-course.

The notion of a validation group is particularly useful to the practitioner–researcher, who is often working on her own, and serves to counter what Hart (1996) saw as the danger of action research being implicated in a divide-and-rule strategy by managers, and of what Elliott (1991) identified as the tendency of action research to concentrate on individual technical improvements rather than on group efforts to change and innovate.

The validation group also helps to address the emphasis placed by many writers on the collaborative nature of action research, since it enables the practitioner–researcher to focus on ways of improving her own individual practice while at the same time collaborating with a group of peers, managers and patients.

Data analysis

We have already seen that data collection methods in reflexive action research can range from the formal, well-established qualitative and quantitative social research methods to the rather looser and less-recognized methods of reflective diaries and unstructured observations. Clearly, where recognized methods are employed to collect the data, there will usually also be well-established procedures for their analysis. On the other hand, little attention has been paid in the past to the analysis of data collected from reflective diaries or critical incidents.

It must be remembered, however, that the purpose of data analysis in reflexive action research is not primarily to build theory, but to evaluate practice, and the same degree of rigor required of traditional social research is therefore not necessary. Indeed, the evaluation of the effectiveness of practice is often a matter of professional judgement, of whether the practitioner–researcher and her validation group agree that her intervention has resulted in a clinical improvement.

Thus, in the earlier counselling example of AEU research, the analysis of data is simply the practitioner–researcher's subjective judgement that the patient is now talking more and is generally making progress. Similarly, in the introspective example of AEU research the data analysis is the practitioner–researcher's own subjective reflection on whether her intervention has helped the situation. Furthermore, in the family therapy example, it is not the nurse but the clients who analyse the data; in this case the parents of the identified patient, who make a subjective judgement about whether the situation has improved.

Inevitably, many traditional researchers will criticize this approach to analysis as lacking in rigor and objectivity, and of course they are correct. But then rigor and objectivity are not the goals of PCR, as a quick glance back at Table 3.1 will confirm. There will always be problems of subjectivity, of the practitioner–researcher convincing herself that an improvement has occurred when in fact it has not, or more likely, of not recognizing when an improvement has taken place.

However, as we saw in Chapter 3, true objectivity is impossible even in the hard sciences, and when we try to judge the practitioner–researcher's analysis against some scientific 'objective' judgement of whether a clinical improvement has taken place, we are, in fact, merely comparing two subjective accounts, two different views of an essentially unknowable process. The very notion that there is some objective criterion of clinical improvement which the practitioner–researcher's professional judgement can be measured against is therefore naive and incorrect.

However, although data analysis in reflexive action research might not involve a formal process, a written record is still required, not least for the purpose of validation. This might simply take the form of a reflective diary which recounts the action research process, and as with case-study research, diary writing is as much a process of data analysis as it is of data collection. Nevertheless, the written account of the action research, in whatever form it takes, is always secondary to the action itself; it might be an important step along the way, but the real goal of the reflexive action researcher is to bring about an improvement in practice.

Summary

Action research has developed from Lewin's early work in industrial settings into a diverse group of methodologies with little in common. In nursing, the approach is gaining acceptance, but there is little agreement about what it means, and a distinct lack of a focus or rationale. Several writers have proposed typologies in order to clarify the situation, but they have only added to the confusion by using similar terms for different constructs, and different terms for similar constructs. The only point of general (but not total) agreement seems to be that action research is characterized by a succession of cycles or spirals with the aim of initiating and/or understanding change.

For the practitioner–researcher, whose aim is to integrate research into her everyday practice, a reflexive approach to action research is required. The characteristics of reflexive action research include the requirement that the research is carried out by the practitioner into her own practice; that it brings about direct improvement in the situation being researched; and that it contributes to her personal knowledge and theory. Research questions for reflexive action research are thus invariably developmental or 'how?' questions.

Reflexive action research is therefore very different from most other approaches, and requires its own typology. The one developed in this chapter is based around a systems approach to problem solving, and employs different sequences of action, evaluation and understanding in order to break the vicious circle of positive feedback where an attempted solution to a problem actually makes that problem worse.

Three possible research designs are described. First, the UAE design, which is similar to the traditional action research model. In UAE action research, a theory is developed, action is implemented to test the theory, and an evaluation of the action (and hence, of the theory) is carried out. Action is therefore informed and directed by theory. In AEU action research, the action comes first and a theory or understanding develops as a result of evaluating the action. Theory therefore emerges from action. In EUA action research, the research comes first, and the theory and understanding which arises from the research findings is employed to direct the action. Action is therefore informed by research.

As might be expected from an approach which places the emphasis on the action rather than on the research, data collection is not the most important consideration of reflexive action research, and can range from formal scientific methods to informal introspection and reflection. This emphasis on action rather than on theory is also evident in the approach to validity, which focuses on the effectiveness of the practice intervention rather than on the accuracy of the research findings. Reflexive action research is therefore the ultimate utilitarian approach for the practitioner–researcher, since it brings together research and practice as a single process in which she can constantly monitor and refine her clinical work in a reflexive spiral.

Notes for Chapter 6

1. Frankl beautifull illustrated the use of paradoxical intention with a joke:

> A boy who came to school late excused himself to the teacher on the grounds that the icy streets were so slippery that whenever he moved one step forward he slipped two back again. Thereupon the teached retorted, "Now I have caught you in a lie – if this were true, how did you ever get to school?" Whereupon the boy calmly replied, "I finally turned around and went home!"
> (Frankl, 1973)

Sometimes, the best way to get to where we want to be is to go in the opposite direction.

REFLECTIVE BREAK

DESIGNING REFLEXIVE ACTION RESEARCH

Turn back to the environmental practice-based development question that you formulated in the Reflective Break on page 93. Outline a reflexive action research project to answer that question under the following headings:

Problem to be addressed (e.g. what is the problem for *you* in *your* practice?)

Personal interest and prejudice in the problem

Research question (from Reflective Break on page 93)

Research design (including statements about the understanding, action and evaluation phases in the appropriate sequence)

Why is this design most appropriate for your research?

Data collection methods

Ethical and practical constraints

Expected outcomes

2. Indeed, the nursing process can be seen as a form of UAE action research in which a theoretical assessment is carried out, a nursing action is implemented, and an evaluation is made of its effectiveness.

Epilogue

Towards a critical community

Part One of this book attempted to explore the epistemology of nursing practice and offered a model of how different kinds of knowing could be combined in a clinical problem-solving strategy which draws on the nurse's expertise and professional judgement as much as on her technical and scientific knowledge. One of the implications of such a model is that scientific research is, by itself, inadequate for the task of informing clinical decisions, and the only way that nurses can acquire the relevant research-based knowledge is to carry out research for themselves into their own practice. Part Two of this book took up the challenge of developing a paradigm of practitioner-centred research (PCR), and identified three methodologies to meet three very distinct needs of the practitioner-researcher.

First, the practitioner-researcher needs to be able to verify the findings of generalizable scientific research for her own practice with her own patients, and to begin to map out the uses and limitations of scientific knowledge when applied to individual cases. In other words, she needs a way of turning generalizable scientific theory into specific personal theory and knowledge. This involves not only the testing of published research findings in the practitioner-researcher's own clinical area with her own patients, but also extending those findings to new situations.

I have called this approach to PCR *replicative research*, and I identified and discussed the methodology of single-case experimental research (SCER) as a particularly appropriate way of doing it. SCER offers a systematic approach to evaluating different interventions on single subjects, and by careful selection of cases, the limits and boundaries of the effectiveness of those interventions can be mapped out. Thus, when the practitioner-researcher uses SCER to replicate a published study in her own clinical area with her own patients, she is not replicating the method, but rather she is attempting to reproduce the findings in order to determine in which situations and with which patients those findings are of use, and in which situations and with which patients they are not.

Secondly, the practitioner–researcher needs to generate her own personal knowledge and theories in her own practice setting and with her own patients. But as we saw from Part One of this book, personal knowledge is not only knowledge about the individuals we are working with, but more importantly it is knowledge about ourselves, about our attitudes, knowledge and skills, and about the effectiveness of our clinical interventions. What is required is therefore a reflective approach to PCR, an approach in which the practitioner–researcher can examine herself and her own impact on the clinical situation she is involved in.

I have referred to this approach to PCR as *reflective research*, and I have outlined and explored a modified form of case study and/or ethnography as its principal methodology. However, unlike tradi-tional approaches, reflective case-study research is overtly subjective and inward-looking rather than objective and outward-looking, and employs reflection on our own participation in our own practice as the primary data collection method, supported by and triangulated with a variety of more usual case-study methods.

Finally, the practitioner–researcher needs to be able to integrate research into her everyday practice such that her practice is reflexively shaped and driven by an ongoing evaluation of her actions and their consequences. I have referred to this as *reflexive research*, and I have offered a modified form of action research based around a systems approach to problem-solving as the most appropriate way of doing it.

Together, I have suggested that these three methodologies provide an alternative paradigm for doing clinical research, a paradigm which provides knowledge and theory that is of direct use to the practitioner for the simple reason that it is generated by the practitioner from her work with her own patients (Table A). Furthermore, it is an approach to research which values subjectivity and the practice perspective, which appeals to professional judgement rather than to scientific method as the basis for clinical decisions, and which is concerned primarily with the development of practice rather than with the discovery of scientific knowledge. In short, it is an attempt to value the practice-based personal and experiential knowledge of the practitioner above the theory-based scientific knowledge of the academic researcher

Table A.   A summary of the principal methodologies of PCR

	Replicative research	Reflective research	Reflexive research
Principal methodology	Single-case experiments	Reflective case study	Reflexive action research
Functions	Local verification of scientific research findings; verification of own personal and experiential knowledge; construction and development of practice-based theories; comparision of the effectiveness of clinical interventions	Description of clinical situations; understanding of ourselves and our practice; formulation and testing of theories	Improvement of the practice situation; generation of personal theory; integration of research and practice
Research questions	Descriptive	Usually exploratory	Developmental
Methods	Quantitative	Triangulation of mostly qualitative methods	Qualitative or quantitative, depending on the the practice setting to be evaluated

Towards a critical community

One of the biggest problems with PCR as I have outlined it in this book is that of sharing our findings with others. The difficulty in working outside of the dominant paradigm is that the guardians and upholders of the paradigm are unlikely to accept our work as a valid contribution to the knowledge-base of the discipline. We have already seen that the Department of Health rejects small-scale non-generalizable projects and has called for them to be curbed, and PCR is therefore very unlikely to attract major funding. However, this is of little consequence to most practitioner-researchers because PCR is comparatively cheap to carry out, and is often done as part of normal, everyday clinical practice.

What is more problematical, however, is the attempt to share the findings of PCR with a wider audience, since most academic and professional journal and conference review panels would reject them as methodologically unsound when judged against the criteria of the technical rationality paradigm. Furthermore, it has also been pointed out that PCR can be a very lonely and potentially isolating experience, and that 'in the act of self-reflection the subject can deceive itself' (Habermas, 1974). Practitioner–researchers must therefore seek forums other than the traditional academic outlets for sharing the experiences and findings of their research.

One such way is through forming 'critical communities' of like-minded practitioner–researchers for sharing, validating and evaluating PCR. Carr and Kemmis (1986) referred to these as 'self-reflective communities' and McNiff (1993) used the term 'dialogical communities' comprising 'peer-practitioners who are concerned to move each others understanding of practice forward by engaging in dialogue'.

Van Manen (1990) echoed this description, claiming that the aim of such communities should be 'collaborative discussions' or 'herme-neutic conversations' which are aimed not only at sharing our work, but at 'generating deeper insights and understandings', what Gadamer (1975) described as 'the art of testing'. This testing or questioning is not intended to outwit or trick the other person, however, but rather:

> the structure of the conversational relation much more resembles the dialogic relation of what Socrates called the situation of "talking together like friends". Friends do not try to make the other weak; in contrast, friends aim to bring out strength.
>
> (Van Manen, 1990)

The members of the critical community are therefore critical friends, whose purpose is to direct the naturally introspective focus of PCR outwards 'so that the researcher, working from the information gathered, can begin to perceive new possibilities and developments' (Edwards and Talbot, 1994). A good example of this outward focusing is given by Miller (1990), who cited a teacher talking about being part of a critical support group:

> This group breaks down the isolation for me. I feel as though I am now part of a bigger picture. This gives me a chance to talk and think. I feel so much more confident as a teacher, as I realise that a lot of my

frustration isn't all my fault. I share more readily and I'm not so resistant to others' ideas ... I feel that this group is a bridge, letting me go back and forth from myself and this group to my larger worlds and then back again.

The role of the critical community in bringing practitioner–researchers together and allowing them to contextualize their work in the larger scheme of things introduces a political element, and as Carr and Kemmis (1986) pointed out, this

offers a first step to overcoming aspects of the existing social order which frustrates rational change: it organizes practitioners into collaborative groups for the purposes of their own enlightenment.

Elliott (1991) developed this point further. He claimed that the lone practitioner–researcher lives under the illusion that improvement of practice is largely a matter of developing technical skills, whereas this illusion is, in fact, the product of a deliberate plan to prevent practitioners from seeking 'real' political power. It is, he argued, only by coming together that practitioners can 'develop the courage to critique the ... structures which shape their practices, and the power to negotiate change within the system which maintains them' (Elliott, 1991).

Edwards and Talbot (1994) echoed this sentiment, claiming that 'the process of systematically gathering data about practice is a political one'. They continued:

Well informed practitioners, armed with convincing data and articulate about the significance of elements of practice are able to deal with confidence with a world that is far from cosy. This level of confidence, however, can usually only occur if opportunities for talking about what is happening can be part of the process.

Critical communities therefore have a number of defining characteristics and a number of functions. They are self-critical, supportive, challenging, empowering, non-hierarchical groups which can transcend clinical and professional boundaries. They can serve to overcome feelings of isolation, to validate and extend our findings, to locate our research in the real world, and to organize and empower practitioners for wider political action.

Furthermore, and most importantly, by coming together to share our work in a critical community, we are affirming and validating what we are doing. It might be recalled that PCR was defined earlier as 'systematic self-critical enquiry *made public*', and so sharing the findings from our work with a wider community of practitioners and researchers not only makes a statement about the importance of this sort of research and the practitioners who undertake it, but is essential in establishing its status as a valid form of research.

But we should not think of the critical community simply as a forum for the oral presentation of our research. We have already explored the creative potential of writing, and membership of a critical community must not be seen as an alternative to the task of putting pen to paper (or fingers to keyboard!). Whatever knowledge might arise from doing PCR, it is only by writing and sharing it with others that we can hope to bring about lasting changes to practice.

I concluded a previous book by claiming that no amount of reading will ever make us better practitioners, and that the only books that will really influence our practice are those that we write ourselves. It is only by writing that we come to understand our thoughts and actions, and I hope that this guide to expanding your nursing knowledge through research has encouraged you not only to give some thought to your own practical knowledge-base, but to begin the critical and creative act of writing and sharing it with others.

REFLECTIVE BREAK

BUILDING A CRITICAL COMMUNITY

Critical communities have a wider role than simply sharing PCR. Try to identify a focus for a critical community in your own practice area. It could be a specific clinical issue or a more general area of practice.

Who might contribute to this critical community? Remember that critical communities should be multidisciplinary and non-hierarchical.

What might be the aims of the community?

How could those aims be realized?

References

Adelman, C., Jenkins, D. and Kemmis, S. (1976) 'Re-thinking case study: notes from the second Cambridge conference', *Cambridge Journal of Education*, 6, 139–150.

Aggleton, P. and Chalmers, H. (1986) *Nursing Models and the Nursing Process*, London: Macmillan.

Andrews, H.A. and Roy, C. (1986) *Essentials of the Roy Adaptation Model*, Norwalk: Appleton-Century-Crofts.

Andrews, M. (1996) 'Using reflection to develop clinical expertise', *British Journal of Nursing*, 5, (8), 508–513.

Auden, W.H. (1967) 'A short defense of poetry'. Conference address cited in Van Manen, M. (1990) *Researching Lived Experience*, New York: SUNY.

Baer, D.M. (1977) 'Perhaps it would be better not to know everything', *Journal of Applied Behavior Analysis*, 10, 167–172.

Baer, D.M., Wolf, M.M. and Risley, T.R. (1968) 'Some current dimensions of applied behavior analysis', *Journal of Applied Behavior Analysis*, 1, 91–97.

Bailey, R. and Clarke, M. (1989) *Stress and Coping in Nursing*, London: Chapman and Hall.

Bamberger, J. and Schön, D.A. (1991) 'From research experience to reflexive method: learning as reflective conversation with materials'. In Steier, F. (ed.) *Research and Reflexivity*, London: Sage.

Barlow, D.H. and Hersen, M (1973) 'Single-case experimental designs: uses in applied clinical research', *Archives of General Psychiatry*, 29, 319–325.

Barlow, D.H. and Hersen, M (1984) *Single Case Experimental Designs*, New York: Pergamon.

Barthes, R. (1977) *Image Music Text*, London: Fontana.

Barthes, R. (1986) *The Rustle of Language*, New York: Hill and Wang.

Becker, H.S. (1958) 'Problems of inference and proof in participant observation' *American Sociological Review*, 23, (6), 652–660.

Becker, H.S. (1986) *Writing for Social Scientists*, Chicago: University of Chicago Press.

Benner, P. (1984) *From Novice to Expert*, California: Addison-Wesley.

Benner, P. and Tanner, C. (1987) 'Clinical judgement: how expert nurses use intuition', *American Journal of Nursing*, 87, (1), 23–31.

Benner, P. and Wrubel, J. (1989) *The Primacy of Caring*, California: Addison-Wesley.

Bergin, A.E. (1966) 'Some implications of psychotherapy research for therapeutic practice', *Journal of Abnormal Psychology*, 71, 235–246.

Bergin, A.E. and Strupp, H.H. (1970) 'New directions in psychotherapy research', *Journal of Abnormal Psychology*, 76, 13–26.

Bergin, A.E. and Strupp, H.H. (1972) *Changing Frontiers in the Science of Psychotherapy*, New York: Aldine.

Bines, H. (1992) 'Issues in course design'. In Bines, H. and Watson, D. (eds) *Developing Professional Education*, Buckingham: Open University Press.

Blake, W. (1808) 'Annotations to Sir Joshua Reynold's "Discourses" '. In Keynes, G. (ed) (1959) *Complete Writings*, London: Oxford University Press.

Blumer, H. (1954) 'What is wrong with social theory?', *American Sociological Review*, 19, 3–10.

Boyd, E.M. and Fales, A.W. (1983) 'Reflective learning: key to learning from experience', *Journal of Humanistic Psychology*, 23, (2), 99–117.

Bromley, D. (1986) *The Case-Study Method in Psychology and Related Disciplines*, Chichester: Wiley.

Bruyn, S.T. (1966) *The Human Perspective in Sociology: The method of participant observation*, Englewood Cliffs: Prentice-Hall.

Bullock, A., Stallybrass, O., Trombley, S. and Eadie, B. (eds) (1988) *The Fontana Dictionary of Modern Thought*, London: Harper Collins.

Burgess, R.G. (1984) *In the Field*, London: Routledge.

Burns, N. and Grove, S.K. (1987) *The Practice of Nursing Research*, Philadelphia: W.B. Saunders.

Capra, F. (1976) *The Tao of Physics*, London: Fontana.

Carey, J. (1995) *The Faber Book of Science*, London: Faber and Faber.

Carnap, R. (1970) 'Statistical and inductive probability'. In Brody, B.A. (ed.) *Readings in the Philosophy of Science*, New Jersey: Prentice-Hall.

Carper, B. (1992) 'Philosophical inquiry in nursing: an application'. In Kikuchi, J.F. and Simmons, H. (eds) *Philosophic Inquiry in Nursing*, Newbury Park: Sage.

Carr, W. and Kemmis, S. (1986) *Becoming Critical*, London: Falmer Press.

Chuang Tzu, trans Giles, H.A. (1926) *Chuang Tzu*, London: George Allen and Unwin.

Cicourel, A. (1976) *The Social Organization of Juvenile Justice*, London: Heinemann.

Clarke, B., James, C. and Kelly, J. (1994) 'Reflective practice: broadening the scope' Paper presented to the First International Nursing Times Open Learning Conference, Nottingham.

Clarke, B., James, C. and Kelly, J (1996) 'Reflective practice: reviewing the issues and refocusing the debate', *International Journal of Nursing Studies*, 33, (2), 171–180.

Cohen, L.H. (1976) 'Clinicians utilisation of research findings', *JSAS Catalog of Selected Documents in Psychology*, 6, 116.

Cohen, L and Manion, L. (1985) *Research Methods in Education*, London: Croom Helm.

Corey, S.M. (1953) *Action Research to Improve School Practices*, Columbia: New York Teachers' College.

Cronbach, L.J. (1975) 'Beyond the two disciplines of scientific psychology', *American Psychologist*, 30, 116–127.

Denzin, N.K. (1978) *The Research Act: a theoretical introduction to sociological methods*, New York: McGraw-Hill.

Denzin, N.K. (1997) *Interpretive Ethnography*, London: Sage.

Department of Health (1989) *A Strategy for Nursing: a report of the Steering Committee*, London: DoH.

Department of Health (1993) *Report of the Taskforce on the Strategy for Research in Nursing, Midwifery and Health Visiting*, London: HMSO.

Department of Health (1995) *The Nursing and Therapy Professions' Contribution to Health Services Research and Development*, London: DoH.

Dewey, J. (1938) *Experience and Education*, New York: Macmillan.

Dreyfus, H.L. (1979) *What Computers can't do: the limits of artificial intelligence*, New York: Harper and Row.

Dreyfus, H.L. and Dreyfus, S.E. (1986) *Mind Over Machine*, Oxford: Basil Blackwell.

Ebbutt, D. (1985) 'Educational action research: some general concerns and specific quibbles'. In Burgess, R.G. (ed.) *Issues in Educational Research: qualitative methods*, Lewes: Falmer Press.

Edwards, A. and Talbot, R. (1994) *The Hard-Pressed Researcher*, London: Longman.

Elliott, J. (1976–7) 'Developing hypotheses about classrooms from teachers practical constructs: an account of the work of the Ford Teaching Project', *Interchange*, 7, 2.

Elliott, J. (1978) 'What is action research in schools?', *Journal of Curriculum Studies*, 10, (4), 355–357.

Elliott, J. (1991) *Action Research for Educational Change*, Milton Keynes: Open University Press.

Ellis, C. and Bochner, A.P. (1996) *Composing Ethnography*, London: Alta Mira.

Elstein, A.S. and Bordage, G. (1988) 'Psychology of clinical reasoning'. In Downie, J. and Elstein. A. (eds) *Professional Judgement*, Cambridge: Cambridge University Press.

Eysenck, H. (1965) 'The effects of psychotherapy', *International Journal of Psychiatry*, 1, 97–178.

Feyerabend, P.K. (1970) 'Against method: outline of an anarchistic theory of knowledge', *Minnesota Studies in the Philosophy of Science*, 4, 17–130.

Fitzgerald, M. (1994) 'Theories of reflection for learning'. In Palmer, A., Burns, S. and Bulman, C. (eds) *Reflective Practice in Nursing*, Oxford: Blackwell Scientific.

Frankl, V.E. (1973) *Psychotherapy and Existentialism*, Harmondsworth: Penguin.

Fuller, R. and Petch, A. (1995) *Practitioner Research*, Buckingham: Open University Press.

Gadamer, H.G. (1975) *Truth and Method*, New York: Seabury.

Gadamer, H.G. (1976) *Philosophical Hermeneutics*, California: University of California Press.

Gadamer, H.G. (1996) *The Enigma of Health*, Oxford: Blackwell.

Garfinkel, H. (1967) *Studies in Ethnomethodology*, Englewood Cliffs: Prentice-Hall.

Geertz, C. (1973) *The Interpretation of Cultures*, New York: Basic Books.

Gibbings, S. (1993) 'Informed action', *Nursing Times*, 89, (46), 28–31.

Giorgi, A. (1971) 'Phenomenology and experimental psychology'. In Giorgi, A., Fischer, W.F. and Von Eckartsberg, R. (eds) *Duquesne Studies in Phenomenological Psychology*, Pittsburg: Duquesne University Press.

Glaser, B. and Strauss, A. (1967) *The Discovery of Grounded Theory*, Chicago: Aldine.

Good, D.A. and Watts, F.N. (1989) 'Qualitative Research'. In Parry, G. and Watts, F.N. (eds) *Behavioural and Mental Health Research: a handbook for skills and methods*, Hove: Lawrence Erlbaum.

Gordon, D.R. (1984) 'Research application: identifying the use and misuse of formal models in nursing practice'. In Benner, P. (ed.) *From Novice to Expert*, California: Addison-Wesley.

Greenwood, E. (1966) 'Attributes of a profession'. In H.M. Vollmer and D.L. Mills (eds) *Professionalization*, Englewood Cliffs: Prentice-Hall.

Greenwood, J. (1984) 'Nursing research: a position paper', *Journal of Advanced Nursing*, 9, 77–82.

Greenwood, J. (1994) 'Action research: a few details, a caution and something new', *Journal of Advanced Nursing*, 20, 13–18.

Guba, E. and Lincoln, Y. (1989) *Fourth Generation Evaluation*, Newbury Park: Sage.

Habermas, J. (1974) *Theory and Practice*, London: Heinemann.

Hakim, C. (1987) *Research Design*, London: Unwin Hyman.

Hamilton, D. (1980) 'Some contrasting assumptions about case study research and survey analysis'. In Simons, H. (ed.) *Towards a Science of the Singular*, Norwich: University of East Anglia.

Hammersley, M. (1992) *What's Wrong with Ethnography?*, London: Routledge.

Hammersley, M. and Atkinson, P. (1983) *Ethnography: principles in practice*, London: Routledge.

Harman, G. (1965) 'The inference to the best explanation', *Philosophical Review*, 74, 88–95.

Harris, M. (1968) *The Rise of Anthropological Theory*, New York: Crowell.

Hart, E. (1996) 'Action research as a professionalizing strategy: issues and dilemmas', *Journal of Advanced Nursing*, 23, 454–461.

Hart, E. and Bond, M. (1995) *Action Research for Health and Social Care*, Buckingham: Open University Press.

Hartley, J.F. (1994) 'Case studies in organizational research'. In Cassell, C. and Symon, G. (eds) *Qualitative Methods in Organizational Research*, London: Sage.

Hayes, S.C. (1981) 'Single case experimental design and empirical clinical practice', *Journal of Consulting and Clinical Psychology*, 49, 193–211.

Heisenberg, W. (1963) *Physics and Philosophy*, London: Allen and Unwin.

Hicks, C. (1996) 'A study of nurses attitudes towards research: a factor analytic approach', *Journal of Advanced Nursing*, 23, 373–379.

Holter, I.M. and Schwartz-Barcott, D. (1993) 'Action research: what is it? How has it been used and how can it be used in nursing?', *Journal of Advanced Nursing*, 18, 298–304.

Hughes, J. (1990) *The Philosophy of Social Research*, London: Longman.

Hunt, J. (1982) 'The recognition battle', *Nursing Mirror*, 154, (9), March 3, 24–26.

International Council of Nurses (1996) *Better Health Through Nursing Research*, Geneva: ICN.

Janes, R.W. (1961) 'A note on the phases of the community role of the participant observer', *American Sociological Review*, 26, (3), 446–450.

Jarvis, P. (1983) *Professional Education*, London: Croom Helm.

Josephson, J.R. and Josephson, S.G. (1994) *Abductive Inference*, Cambridge: Cambridge University Press.

Kazdin, A.E. (1984) 'Statistical analyses for single-case experimental designs'. In Barlow, D.H. and Hersen, M. (eds) *Single Case Experimental Designs*, New York: Pergamon.

Kalleberg, R. (1990) *The Construct Turn in Sociology*, Oslo: Institute for Social Research.

Kemmis, S. (1980) 'The imagination of the case and the invention of the study'. In Simons, H. (ed.) *Towards a Science of the Singular*, Norwich: University of East Anglia.

Kemmis, S. (1982) *The Action Research Reader*, Australia: Deaking University Press.

Kemmis, S. and McTaggart, R. (1982) *The Action Research Planner*, Australia: Deakin University Press.

Kerlinger, F.N. (1964) *Foundations of Behavioural Research*, New York: Holt, Rinehart and Winston.

Kiesler, D.J. (1971) 'Experimental designs in psychotherapy research'. In Bergin, A.E. and Garfield, S.L. (eds) *Handbook of Psychotherapy and Behavior Change: an empirical analysis* (2nd edn), New York: Wiley.

Kitwood, T.M. and Bredin, K. (1994) *Evaluating Dementia Care: the DCM method*, Bradford: Bradford Dementia Research Group.

Koch, T. (1994) 'Establishing rigour in qualitative research: the decision trail', *Journal of Advanced Nursing*, 19, 976–986.

Kosko, B. (1994) *Fuzzy Thinking*, London: Harper Collins.

Kuhn, T. (1962) *The Structure of Scientific Revolutions*, Chicago: University of Chicago Press.

Lathlean, J. and Farnish, S. (1984) *The Ward Sister Training Project: An evaluation of a training scheme for ward sisters*, London: University of London Nursing Education Research Unit.

Leitenberg, H. (1973) 'The use of single-case methodology in psychotherapy research', *Journal of Abnormal Psychology*, 82, 87–101.

Lewin, K. (1946) 'Action research and minority problems', *Journal of Social Issues*, 2, 34–46.

Lewin, K. (1948) *Resolving Social Conflicts*, New York: Harper.

Lofland, J. (1970) 'Interactionist imagery and analytic interrurtus'. In Shibutani, T. (ed.) *Human Nature and Collective Behaviour*, Englewood Cliffs: Prentice-Hall.

Lofland, J. and Lofland, L. (1984) *Analysing Social Settings: A guide to qualitative observation and analysis*, Belmont: Wadsworth.

MacDonald, B. (1980) 'Letters from a headmaster'. In Simons, H. (ed.) *Towards a Science of the Singular*, Norwich: University of East Anglia.

Macleod Clark, J. and Hockey, L. (1989) *Further Research for Nursing*, London: Scutari.

MacGuire, J. (1991) 'Tailoring research for advanced nursing practice'. In McMahon, R. and Pearson, A. (eds) *Nursing as Therapy*, London: Chapman and Hall.

McKernan, J. (1991) *Curriculum Action Research*, London: Kogan Page.
McNiff, J. (1993) *Teaching as Learning*, London: Routledge.
McNiff, J., Lomax, P. and Whitehead, J. (1996) *You and Your Action Research Project*, London: Routledge.
Malinowski, B. (1922) *Argonauts of the Western Pacific*, London: Routledge and Kegan Paul.
Maxwell, N. (1984) *From Knowledge to Wisdom: a revolution in the aims and methods of science*, Oxford: Blackwell.
May, T. (1993) *Social Research*, Buckingham: Open University Press.
Merton, R.K. (1968) *Social Theory and Social Structure*, New York: Free Press.
Miller, J. (1990) *Creating Spaces and Finding Voices*, New York: SUNY.
Mills, C.W. (1959) *The Sociological Imagination*, Harmondsworth: Penguin.
Milne, A.A. (1926) *Winnie-the-Pooh*, London: E.P. Dutton.
Morley, S. (1989) 'Single case research'. In Parry, G. and Watts, F.N. (eds) *Behavioural and Mental Health Research: a handbook for skills and methods*, Hove: Lawrence Erlbaum.
Morse, J. M. (1991) *Qualitative Nursing Research*, London: Sage.
Nisbet, J. and Watt, J. (1979) *Case Study*, Nottingham: Rediguide.
Pallis, D.J., Gibbons, J.S. and Pierce, D.W. (1984) 'Estimating suicide risk among attempted suicides', *British Journal of Psychiatry*, 144, 139–148.
Peck, D.F. (1989) 'Research with single (or few) patients'. In Freeman, C. and Tyrer, P. (eds) *Research Methods in Psychiatry*, London: Gaskell.
Platt, J. (1981) 'On interviewing one's peers', *British Journal of Sociology*, 32, (1), 75–91.
Polanyi, M. (1962) *Personal Knowledge: towards a post-critical philosophy*, London: Routledge and Kegan Paul.
Polit, D.F. and Hungler, B.P. (1991) *Nursing Research: principles and methods*, 4th edn, Philadelphia: Lippincott.
Popper, K. (1979) *Objective Knowledge: an evolutionary approach* revised edn, Oxford: OUP.
Powers, B.A. and Knapp, T.R. (1995) *A Dictionary of Nursing Theory and Research* (2nd edn), London: Sage.
Pryjmachuk, S. (1996) 'A nursing perspective on the interrelationships between theory, research and practice', *Journal of Advanced Nursing*, 23, 679–684.
Radwin, L.E. (1995) 'Knowing the patient: a process model for individualized interventions', *Nursing Research*, 44, (6), 364–370.
Reason, P. (ed.) (1988) *Human Inquiry in Action*, London: Sage.
Reason, P. and Rowan, J. (eds) (1981) *Human Inquiry*, Chichester: Wiley.
Rogers, C.R. (1956) 'A changed view of science'. In Rogers, C.R. (ed.) *On Becoming a Person*, London: Constable.
Rogers, C.R. (1974) *On Becoming a Person*, London: Constable.
Rolfe, G. (1993) 'Closing the theory–practice gap: a model of nursing praxis', *Journal of Clinical Nursing*, 2, 173–177.
Rolfe, G. (1996) *Closing the Theory Practice Gap: a new paradigm for nursing*, Oxford: Butterworth Heinemann.
Ryle, G. (1963) *The Concept of Mind*, Harmondsworth: Penguin.
Sandelowski, M. (1986) 'The problem of rigor in qualitative research', *Advances in Nursing Science*, 8, 27.

Sanford, N. (1970) 'Whatever happened to action research?', *Journal of Social Issues*, **26**, 3–13.

Sapsford, R. and Abbott, P. (1992) *Research Methods for Nurses and the Caring Professions*, Milton Keynes: Open University Press.

Schatzman, L. and Strauss, A. (1973) *Field Research: strategies for a natural sociology*, Englewood Cliffs: Prentice-Hall.

Schlipp, P.A. (1948) *Albert Einstein, Philosopher-Scientist*, Evanston, Illinois: Tudor.

Schön, D.A. (1983) *The Reflective Practitioner*, London: Temple Smith.

Schön, D.A. (1987) *Educating the Reflective Practitioner*, San Francisco: Jossey-Bass.

Schramm, W. (1971) *Notes on Case Studies of Instructional Media Projects*, Washington, DC: Academy for Educational Development.

Schutz, S.E. (1994) 'Exploring the benefits of a subjective approach in qualitative nursing research', *Journal of Advanced Nursing*, **20**, 412–417.

Shipman, M.D. (1972) *The Limitations of Social Research*, London: Longman.

Shontz, F.C. (1965) *Research Methods in Personality*, New York: Appleton-Century-Crofts.

Slevin, O. and Basford, L. (eds) (1995) *Theory and Practice of Nursing*, Edinburgh: Campion Press.

Sparrow, S. and Robinson, J. (1994) 'Action research: an appropriate design for nursing research?', *Educational Action Research*, **2**, (3), 347–356.

Stake, R. (1980) 'The case study method in social inquiry'. In Simons, H. (ed.) *Towards a Science of the Singular*, Norwich: University of East Anglia.

Stenhouse, L. (1975) *An Introduction to Curriculum Research and Development*, London: Heinemann.

Stenhouse, L. (1977) 'Teachers for all seasons', *British Journal of Teacher Education*, **3**, 3.

Stenhouse, L. (1978) 'Case study and case records: towards a contemporary history of education', *British Educational Research Journal*, **4**, (2), 21–39.

Stenhouse, L. (1979a) 'Using research means doing research'. In Dahl, H., Lysne, A. and Rand, P. (eds) *Spotlight on Educational Problems*, Oslo: Oslo University Press.

Stenhouse, L. (1979b) 'The problem of standards in illuminative research', *Scottish Educational Review*, **11**, (1), 5–10.

Stenhouse, L. (1981) 'What counts as research?' *British Journal of Educational Studies*, **29**, (2), 103–114.

Stenhouse, L. (1984a) 'A note on case study and educational practice'. In Burgess, R.G. (ed.) *Field Methods in the Study of Education*, London: Falmer Press.

Stenhouse, L. (1984b) 'Artistry and teaching: the teacher as the focus of research and development'. In Hopkins, D. and Wideen, M. (eds) *Alternative Perspectives on School Improvement*, London: Falmer Press.

Stenhouse, L. (1985a) 'The psycho-statistical paradigm and its limitations'. In Ruddock, J. and Hopkins, D. (eds) *Research as a Basis for Teaching*, Oxford: Heinemann.

Stenhouse, L. (1985b) 'Reporting research to teachers: the appeal to professional judgement'. In Ruddock, J. and Hopkins, D. (eds) *Research as a Basis for Teaching*, Oxford: Heinemann.

Stenhouse, L. (1985c) 'Action research and the teacher's responsibility for the educational process'. In Ruddock, J. and Hopkins, D. (eds) *Research as a Basis for Teaching*, Oxford: Heinemann.

Thompson, J. (1990) 'Hermeneutic inquiry'. In Moody, E. (ed.) *Advancing Nursing Science through Research*, Vol 2, Newbury Park: Sage.

Truzzi, M. (1983) 'Sherlock Holmes: applied social psychologist'. In Eco, U. and Sebeok, T.A. (eds) *The Sign of Three: dupin, holmes, peirce*, Bloomington: Indiana University Press.

Usher, R. and Bryant, I. (1989) *Adult Education as Theory, Practice and Research*, London: Routledge.

Van Manen, M. (1990) *Researching Lived Experience*, New York: State University of New York Press.

Van Manen, M. (1991) *The Tact of Teaching*, New York: State University of New York Press.

Watson, J.B. (1925) *Behaviourism*, London: Kegan Paul.

Webb, C. (1989) 'Action research: philosophy, methods and personal experiences', *Journal of Advanced Nursing*, **14**, 403–410.

Webb, C. (1990) 'Partners in research', *Nursing Times*, **86**, (32), 40–44.

Weller, B.F. (ed.) (1989) *Baillière's Encyclopaedic Dictionary of Nursing and Health Care*, London: Baillière Tindall.

Williams, R. and Morgan, H.G. (1994) *Suicide Prevention: the challenge confronted*, London: HMSO.

Winter, R. (1987) *Action-Research and the Nature of Social Inquiry*, Aldershot: Avebury.

Wolcott, H. (1990) *Writing Up Qualitative Research*, London: Sage.

Wright, S. (1992) In Butterworth, T. and Faugier, J. (eds) *Clinical Supervision and Mentorship in Nursing*, London: Chapman and Hall.

Yin, R.K. (1994) *Case Study Research*, 2nd edn, London: Sage.

Index

Page numbers printed in **bold** type refer to figures; those in *italic* to tables

ABAB designs and variations, in single-case experimental research, 105–6, 106–11, 125

Abduction (abductive reasoning), 47–8, 48–9, 64

Academic validation, 193

Action-evaluation-understanding (AEU) research design, 184–6, 189, 196

Action research *see* Reflexive action research

Agriculture, psycho-statistical paradigm in, 23–4

Analysis *see* Data analysis

Analysis units, case-study research, 135–7

Analytic (logical) generalization, 79–81, 101
   see also Analytic induction

Analytic induction
   reflective case-study research, 164–5
   see also Analytic (logical) generalization

Anticipative reflection, 43, 63

Apprenticeship, acquiring of knowledge, 2, 28

Archives, case-study research, 143–4

Attitudinal measures, in single-case experimental research, 118–19, 120

Authority and validity, case-study research, 161–2

Behavioural measures, 119, 149

Benner, Patricia, 27, 28–30, 34–6, 40–1
   model of expertise, 51–2

Broca, Paul, 102

Case-study research *see* Reflective case-study research

Casualties, in standardized procedures, 23–4

Chance *see* Probability

Chicago School of Ethnography, 127

Circumstances of case-study research, 162

Client validation, 193

Clinical problems, systems approach, 179–80

Clinical supervision
   original aim, 3
   and practitioner-centred research, 96
   and reflective case-study research, 155

Collaboration, 202
   in action research, 175, 194

Comparative case studies, 138

Computers
   expert systems, 45–6
   fuzzy logic, 46

Confidentiality, reflective case-study research, 142, 157

Constant comparative method of data analysis, 164

Construct validity, 160

Converging lines of enquiry, 135
Cooperative inquiry school of
    research, 74–5
Creativity, 85–7
Critical communities, 202–4
    characteristics, 203
    functions, 203
    reflective break, 205
Critical incident analysis, 96,
    155
Cybernetics, 179–80

Data analysis
    in action research, 194–5
    case-study research, 162–7
    constant comparative method,
        164
    single-case experimental
        research, 121–4, 125
    validation combined with, 164
Data collection, 13
    in action research, 189–91,
        196
    case-study research, 131–2,
        140–58, 168
    participant observation, 130,
        131–2, 148
    a political process, 203
    single-case experimental
        research, 116–19, 125
    triangulation, 135, 158, 161,
        168
Data recording, scaling, 122–3
DCM (dementia care mapping),
    149–50
Decision-making
    judges and nurses, 46–7
    see also Professional
        judgement
Deduction (deductive reasoning),
    10, 11, 12
Deliberative reflection, 50–1

Dementia care mapping (DCM),
    149–50
Dewey, John, 44–5
Dialogical communities, 202
Direct observation see Non-
    participant observation
Documentation, reflective case-
    study research, 140–3
    access to, 142–3
    bias, 141
    confidentiality, 142
    types of, 140–1
    use of, 141
    see also Records; Reports;
        Writing

Ebinghaus, Hermann, 102
Education
    action research in, 172–3,
        187–8
    by apprenticeship, 2, 28
    teacher as researcher, 173, 187
    technocratic approach, 1–2
Educational laboratories, 58–9
Elitism, 51–2
Epistemology
    of action research, 174–5
    definition, 3
    of nursing, 25–7
    see also Knowledge
Errors
    type I, 39, 124
    type II, 22, 124
Ethnocentrism, 150
Ethnographic observation see
    Participant observation
Ethnography, 73–4
    reflexive, 169
Evaluation-understanding-action
    (EUA) research design,
    186–8, 189, 196
Experience, systemization of, 95

Experiential knowledge, 31, *32*, 36–7, 42, 43
  nurse beginners, 60–3
  practical, *32*, 33, 34
  v. scientific knowledge, 67
  theoretical, *32*, 33
Expert systems, 45–6
Expertise, 30–1
  knowledge for, 34–7
  v. praxis, 52–3
  as unconscious intuition, 51–2

Farming, psycho-statistical paradigm in, 23–4
Feedback loops, 179–80
  reflective break, 181
Fieldnotes, in case-study research, 132
Fittingness, 79
Ford Teaching Project, 172
Fuzzy logic, 46–7

Galileo, 9–12
General public, as validators, 193
Generalizability
  in clinical research, 22
  of experiential knowledge to other situations, 30, 39
  and practitioner-centred research (PCR), 78–82
Generalization
  analytic (logical), 79–81, 101
  general *v.* individual, vii–viii, 11, 15, 19–24, 72
  naturalistic, 79
  of paradigm cases, 78
  statistical, 79, 101

Hawthorne effect, 130
History
  v. ethnography, 73–4
  paradigm of, 72–3, 74

Incidents *see* Critical incident analysis
Induction (inductive reasoning), 10, 11, **12**
  abduction, 47–8, 48–9, 64
  problem of, 16
Inductive probability, 48–9
'Inference to the best explanation', 47, 49, 50
Informal theory, 43
  see also Personal theory
Information giving, 15
'Intellectual craftsmanship', 154
Inter-rater reliability, 109–10, 121
Intersubject variability, 113
Interviews, case-study research, 144–7
  interviewing oneself, 145–6
  latent identities, 146
Intimacy, in case-study research, 162
Intuition, 51–2
Intuitive grasp, 30–1, 51–2

Judgement *see* Professional judgement

Knowledge
  by apprenticeship, 2, 28
  creation *v.* discovery, 85
  from experience, 30–1
  experiential *see* Experiential knowledge
  for expertise, 34–7
  fundamental patterns of knowing, 27
  general *v.* particular, vii–viii
  knowing how and knowing that, 27–30, *32*, 37
  knowing-in-action, 27–8

measures of, in single-case
    experimental research,
    119
nursing, 31, *32*, 32–4
organismic, 34
personal *see* Personal
    knowledge
practical *see* Practical
    knowledge
reflective breaks, 5, 26, 29,
    35–6, 38
and research, 8–12
scientific *see* Scientific
    knowledge
tacit, 28–9
theoretical *see* Theoretical
    knowledge
and theory, 9–12
two worlds of, vii
world 1, 39
world 2, viii, 31, *32*
world 3, vii–viii, 31, *32*, 33
see also Data analysis;
    Data collection;
    Epistemology

Language, in case-study
    research, 162
Latent identities, 146
Lewin, Kurt, 171–3
Likert scale, 119, 120
Logical (analytic) generalization,
    79–81, 101

Mental Nursing Syllabus (1982),
    2
Methodology
    credibility of, 66–7
    v. method, 101
    *see also under specific types of
        research*
Multiple-case research, 138–40

Naturalism, 130
Naturalistic generalization,
    79
Naturalistic research, 103
Non-participant (direct)
    observation
    case-study research, 147–50
    formal and informal activities,
        148
    problems with, 150
Novice practice, 36, 37
Nurse beginners, 60–3
Nurse–practitioners
    gaining experience, 60–3
    as practitioner–researchers,
        viii–ix
    v. researchers, 65–6, 82
Nurses, involvement in research,
    17
Nursing
    as academic discipline, 1, 2
    aim, 99
    as a science, 7
    technical rationality nursing,
        12–13
Nursing process, as form of
    action research, 198
Nursing research
    definitions, 8–9
    goal, 8–9
    levels of, 101
    see also Research
Nursing theory, 42–3

Objectivity, 83, 84
Observation *see* Non-participant
    observation; Participant
    observation
Opinion measures, in
    single-case experimental
    research, 118–19, 120
Opinion polls, 20–1

Organismic knowledge, 34
Outcome research, 103

Paradigm cases, 28–30, 33, 34,
    36
  generalization of, 78
Paradigm of history, 72–3, 74
Paradigms
  definition, 1
  'new', 74–5, 200
  psycho-statistical, 23–4
  scientific, 7–13
  shifts, 1–3
  see also Practitioner-centred
    research; Technical
    rationality
Paradoxical intention, 182, 183,
    196
Participant (ethnographic)
    observation
  data collection, 130, 131–2,
    148
  fieldnotes, 132
  reflective, 155–7
  reflective case-study research,
    150–8
Patients as individuals, 24
PCR *see* Practitioner-centred
    research
Peer validation, 193
Perceptiveness, 50
Personal knowledge, 31, 32,
    36–7, 42
  fittingness, 79
  nurse beginners, 60–3
  practical, 32, 34
  theoretical, 32, 33–4
  transferability, 79
Personal theory, 42–5
  context specific, 58
  developing, 40–9
  logic of, 45–9

practice setting, 56
  and professional judgement,
    49–63
  'purpose', 44–5
  v. scientific theory, 59
  testing, 50
  see also Informal theory
Physiological measures, in
    single-case experimental
    research, 116–18
Place, of case-study research,
    162
Political power, 203
Popper, Karl, vii–viii, 31
Positivist logic, 58
Practical knowledge, 28, *32*
  experiential, *32*, 33, 34
  personal, *32*, 34
  scientific, *32*, 32–3, 34
Practice, formal *v.* informal, 53
Practice, research-based
  dissatisfaction with, 25
  ethical considerations, 24
  problems with, 24
Practitioner-based enquiry, 75
Practitioner-centred research
    (PCR), 68, 75–8
  critical communities, 202–4,
    205
  definition, 75
  dissemination of findings,
    201–2, 203–4
  establishment opposition to,
    100–1
  functions, *201*
  and generalizability, 78–82
  macro *v.* micro theory, 76
  methodologies, 87–8, 92–8,
    201
  outward focusing, 201–4
  questions *see* Research
    questions

reflective research, 92–4, 200, *201*
reflexive cycle, 76
reflexive research, 94, 200, *201*
replicative research, 92, 199–200, *201*
research methods, *201*
v. scientific research, 71–2, 76, 78
subjectivity in, 83–5
summary, 99–101
v. technical rationality, 75–6, 99–100
third parties as data collectors, 149
see also Reflective case-study research; Reflexive action research; Single-case experimental research
Practitioner–researchers
nurse–practitioners as, viii–ix
v. outside researchers, 142–3, 146–7, 155–7, 162
in practitioner-centred research, 75
Practitioners, v. researchers, vii, 17–18, 65–6, 82
Praxis, 51, 182
v. expertise, 52–3
Prejudice, 84–5
reflective break, 86
Probability, 20–2
inductive, 48–9
replication and, 107–8
Problem of induction, 16
Problem solving, systems approach, 179–80
Process research, 103
Professional judgement, 40–1
cyclical process, 50
decision-making, 46–7

model of, 54–60
personal theory and, 49–63
precedence over research?, 67
reflective breaks, 57, 62, 77
v. scientific theory construction, 58
Professionalization, and reflective action research, 173
Project 2000, 2
Propositions, in case-study research, 137–8
Prudence, 50
Psychiatric nursing, paradigm shift, 2
Psycho-statistical paradigm, 23–4

Questions *see* Research questions

Reasoning
abductive, 47–8, 48–9, 64
deductive, **10**, 11, **12**
inductive *see* Induction
Records
archival, 143–4
contractual *v.* actuarial, 141
reflexive action research, 195
see also Documentation; Reports; Writing
Reflection
anticipative, 43, 63
definition, 41
deliberative, 50–1
original aim, 3
Reflection-in-action, 42, 98
and professional judgement, 53, 55
in reflexive action research, 182

Reflection-on-action, 41–2, 96–7
  and professional judgement,
    52–3, 55
  in reflective case-study
    research, 151, 152
  in reflexive action research,
    185
Reflective breaks
  critical communities, 205
  feedback, 181
  knowledge, 5, 26, 29, 35–6,
    38
  practitioner-centred research
    questions, 93
  prejudice, 86
  professional judgement, 57,
    62, 77
  reflective case-study design,
    170
  reflective writing, 156
  reflexive action research
    design, 197
  scientific research,
    verification, 117
  scientific theory, 14
  single-case experimental
    research project design,
    126
Reflective case-study research,
  95–7, *201*
  analysis units, 135–7
  analytic induction, 164–5
  archival records, 143–4
  authority and validity, 161–2
  comparative case study, 138
  confidentiality, 142, 157
  converging lines of enquiry,
    135
  data analysis, 162–7
  data collection, 131–2,
    140–58, 168
  definitions, 128–9

design, reflective break, 170
  documentation, 140–3
  fieldnotes, 132
  historical development, 127–8
  interviews, 144–7
  methodology, 135–40
  non-participant (direct)
    observation, 147–50
  participant (ethnographic)
    observation, 150–8
  propositions, 137–8
  psychological roots, 127
  reflexivity, 131–2
  reliability, 158–60
  replication model, 139
  reports, 166–7, 169
  research design, 135–40
  research questions, 132–4
  single- and multiple-case
    research, 138–40
  sociological roots, 127
  subjective adequacy, 162
  summary, 167–8
  v. traditional, 136–7
  triangulation in, 135, 158,
    161, 168
  typology development,
    164–5
  uses, 167–8
  validity, 147, 158, 159,
    160–2
  validity maximization, 162
  weaknesses of, 129–31
Reflective diaries, 96
Reflective practice *see*
  Reflection-on-action
Reflective research, 92–4, 200,
  201
Reflective writing, reflective
  break, 156
Reflexive action research, 97–8,
  201

action-evaluation-
    understanding (AEU)
    design, 184–6, 189, 196
aims, 174
characteristics, 178
collaboration, 175, 194
cyclical process, 175
data analysis, 194–5
data collection, 189–91, 196
definitions, 174–6, 179
designing, reflective break,
    197
in education, 172–3, 187–8
epistemology, 174–5
evaluation-understanding-
    action (EUA) design,
    186–8, 189, 196
historical development, 171–4
methodology, 177–89
in nursing, 173–4, 188, 195
reflective model, 173
reliability, 192
research design, 177–89
research questions, 176–7
summary, 195–6
typologies, 177–9
understanding-action-
    evaluation (UAE) design,
    180–4, 189, 196
validity, 191–4
written records, 195
see also Reflection-in-action
Reflexive ethnography, 169
Reflexive practice *see* Reflection-
    in-action
Reflexive research, 94, 200,
    201
Reflexivity, and reflective case-
    study research, 131, 131–2
Reliability
    case-study research, 158–60
    reflexive action research, 192

single-case experimental
    research, 120–1
Replication
    chance results, 107–8
    of studies, 80–1
Replication research model, 139
Replicative research, 92,
    199–200, *201*
Reports
    case-study research, 166–7,
        169
    see also Writing
Research
    action research *see* Reflexive
        action research
    application to practice, 18–19
    artistic approach, 85
    case-studies *see* Reflective
        case-study research
    clinical *v.* theoretical, 63
    comparative case studies, 138
    cooperative inquiry school,
        74–5
    credibility of methodology,
        66–7
    design components, 135
    elitist system, 24
    generalizability, vii–viii, 22
    and knowledge, 8–12
    macro and micro levels, 19–25
    multiple-case, 138–40
    naturalistic, 103
    nursing *see* Nursing research
    outcome research, 103
    percentage probability, 21–2
    practitioner-centred *see*
        Practitioner-centred
        research
    process research, 103
    questions *see* Research
        questions
    reflective, 92–4, 200, *201*

reflexive, 94, 200, *201*
replication model, 139
replicative, 92, 199–200, *201*
rules as guidance, 85–8
sample heterogeneity, 22–3
scientific *see* Scientific
  research
single-case *see* Single-case
  experimental research
soft *v.* hard, 8
supervision of, 157–8
see also Data analysis; Data
  collection
Research act, 68, 85
Research questions, 88–92, *201*
action research *see* reflexive
  action research *below*
case-study research, 132–4,
  136–7
descriptive, 88, 104, 132–3
developmental, 89, 104, 176
environmental, 90, 134, 177
examples, 91–2
explanatory, 133
exploratory, 88–9, 132, 133
focus of, 89, 104, 133, 176
form of, 88–9, 104, 133,
  176
introspective, 89, 133–4,
  136–7, 176
organizational, 89, 104, 133,
  176
personal, 90, 176
practice-based, 89, 104, 133,
  176
reflective break, 93
reflexive action research,
  176–7
single-case experimental
  research, 103–5
subject of, 89–92, 104, 134,
  176–7

Researchers
influence on case studies,
  130–1, 131, 133
as members of researched
  organization, 142–3,
  146–7, 155–7, 162
power of, 17–18
practitioner–researchers,
  viii–ix, 75
v. practitioners, vii, 17–18,
  65–6, 82
Respondent validation, 160–1

SCER *see* Single-case
  experimental research
Science
hard *v.* soft, 7–8
nursing as, 7
pure *v.* applied, 17
'Science of the singular', 72
Scientific knowledge, 31, *32*
v. experiential knowledge, 67
nurse beginners, 60–3
practical, *32*, 32–3, 34
theoretical, *32*, 32
Scientific paradigm, 7–13
Scientific research
aim, 68
and knowledge, 8–12
macro and micro levels, 19–25
nurses' responsibilities, 65–6
and nursing practice, 17–19
v. practitioner-centred research
  (PCR), 71–2, 76, 78
reflective break, 117
subjectivity and prejudice in,
  82–5
see also Research
Scientific theory
constructing and using, **10, 12**
definition, 9
functions of, 10–11, 13

general *v.* individual, 11, 15, 19–24, 72
influence on practice, 11–12
and knowledge, 9–12
limitations, reflective break, 14
v. non-scientific, 9
v. personal theory, 59
proof *v.* disproof, 11
reflective break, 14
Self-awareness, 53
Self-reflective communities, 202
Self-validation, 193
Sensitizing concepts, 164
Single-case experimental research (SCER), 95, 98, 138, 140, 199–200, *201*
ABAB designs and variations, 105–6, 106–11, 125
alternating treatment designs, 106, 113–14, 125
baseline phase length, 115
data analysis, 121–4, 125
data collection methods, 116–19, 125
design approaches, 105–16, 125
design issues, miscellaneous, 114–16
experimental evaluation criterion, 122
historical development, 102–3
inter-rater reliability, 109–10, 121
measures of attitude and opinion, 118–19, 120
measures of behaviour, 119
measures of knowledge, 119
methodology, 105–16
multiple baseline designs, 106, 111–12, 125

physiological measures, 116–18
project design, reflective break, 126
reliability, 120–1
research questions, 103–5
summary, 124–5
test-retest reliability, 121
therapeutic evaluation criterion, 121–2
treatment phase length, 115–16
treatment type variation, 116
uses, 104, 124
validity, 119–20
Situational verification, 92
Social consensus, in case-study research, 162
Statistical generalization, 79, 101
Stenhouse, Lawrence, 65, 66–8, 172
Subjective adequacy, 162
Subjectivity, 82–5
Substantive acts, 68
Suicide risk, 15–16, 22
Supervision
clinical *see* Clinical supervision
of research, 157–8
Systemization of experience, 95

Tavistock Institute of Human Relations, 172, 173
Teaching, aim, 99
Technical rationality, 12–13
alternatives, 25–37
limitations, 13–25
v. practitioner-centred research (PCR), 75–6, 99–100

Technical rationality nursing, 12–13
Test-retest reliability, single-case experimental research, 121
'Textual labor', 152, 153
Theoretical knowledge, 32
    experiential, 32, 33
    personal, 32, 33–4
    scientific, 32, 32
Theories-in-use, 43–4
Theory
    informal, 43
    and knowledge, 9–12
    macro *v.* micro, 76
    nursing, 42–3
    personal *see* Personal theory
    scientific *see* Scientific theory
    testing, 164–5
    types, 9
    of the unique, 72
Theory–practice gap, 15–19, 36, 56, 61, 63
Time, in case-study research, 162
Treatment, single-case experimental research
    ABAB designs and variations, 105–6, 106–11
    phase length, 115–16
    sequential confounding, 113
    variation in type, 116
Triangulation, 135, 158, 161, 168

Understanding-action-evaluation (UAE) research design, 180–4, 189, 196
Unpredictability, 21
Up-liner validation, 193

Validation
    combined with analysis, 164
    interim assessment, 193
    by inviting critiques, 192
    judging core elements of, 192–3
    respondent validation, 160–1
Validation groups, 193–4
Validity
    action research, 191–4
    case-study research, 147, 158, 159, 160–2
    reader's recognition of, 161–2
    single-case experimental research, 119–20

World 1, 39
World 2 knowledge, viii, 31, 32
World 3 knowledge, vii–viii, 31, 32, 33
Writing
    as generator of knowledge, 165–6
    reflective break, 156
    in reflective case-study research, 152–5
    see also Reports